# Gentle Roads
## to Survival

# Gentle Roads
to
# Survival

### Making Self-Healing Choices
### in Difficult Circumstances

by
Andre Auw, Ph.D.

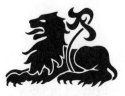

Aslan Publishing

Published by

Aslan Publishing
PO Box 108
Lower Lake, CA 95457

For a free catalog of our other titles,
or to order more copies of this book,
please call (800) 275-2606

**Library of Congress Cataloging-in-Publication Data:**

Auw, André, 1923-
    Gentle roads to survival: making self-healing choices in difficult
circumstances/ by André Auw.
    p.    cm.

    ISBN 0-944031-18-8 : $9.95
    1. Counseling--Miscellanea.  2. Counselors--Psychology.  3. Life
change events--Psychological aspects. 4. Auw, André, 1923-    I. Title.
    BF637.C6A838   1991
    158'. 1--dc20
                                                              90-48311
                                                              CIP

Copyright © 1991, Andre Auw

Cover design by Brenda Plowman
Book design by Dawson Church
Printed in USA
First Edition

10  9  8  7  6  5  4  3  2

To Carl Rogers, mentor and dear friend,
who not only lifted his lamp for me along the dark road,
but permitted me to do the same for him.

# CONTENTS

# Introduction

I was eight years old on a Christmas morning when I saw that beautiful object standing next to the Christmas tree. It was a stunning silver two-wheeled bicycle, brand new, and it was for me. I shall never forget my feelings of surprised joy, nor the thrill of my first ride.

I set out for the foothills nearby, pumping hard, my face stung by the sharp December air. Soon I was coasting downhill at what seemed like record breaking speed. I felt free and powerful. No longer would I be dependent on adults to take me places. Like older boys, I could go wherever my heart desired. My bicycle provided an exciting passage from childhood into boyhood.

Now, from the vantage point of mid-life I realize that I am not alone in valuing the significance of a bicycle for a young boy. Many men I have counseled have recalled with affection memories of their first big bicycle. They remembered the delight of being able to ride without touching the handle bars, of hopping on the bicycle to escape household chores. They spoke of risks and spills, and bumps and bruises as a small price willingly paid in exchange for the rewards received. For them also, a bicycle became a trusted friend, a collaborator in secret adventures, a builder of self confidence, a giver of joy.

At the same time many of these men felt a touch of sadness as they shared their recollections. Like a cloud covering the sun, their yearning for the simplicity of boyhood days dimmed the memory of early joys. It seemed that when they gave up their bicycles and moved into adult life their beliefs changed. As boys they had believed in the limitless capacity to become great, to create new experiences, to overcome huge obstacles. They had confidence in their ability to dream wonderful dreams and to make these dreams come true. They believed it was possible to find rich fulfillment from simple pleasures, even from bicycle riding.

Fear altered these basic beliefs. Counseling often aided in restoring them. The counseling relationship provided a save haven where beliefs could be re-evaluated and fears could be diminished. New feelings of inner strength could join with old memories of self-confidence to build a better belief system. It was as if both persons in the counseling relationship returned to a part of the past and recaptured its power. In spirit, we hopped on our bikes and renewed our belief in ourselves and our power to make our lives significant and satisfying.

This book may offer you similar reminders for your own life experience. It may help you to return to your past and to reclaim your true inner power. Hopefully these chapters will serve to deepen your belief that you can create a fulfilling life, that you can meet challenges with courage, that you have the wisdom to make the best choices possible, that you can prevail over fears that arise to terrify you. And finally, how wonderful to discover that you know the secret to enjoy, amidst all of life's painful periods, the gift of inner peace.

CHAPTER ONE

# *Pushing Away the Clouds*

A few years ago I was traveling on the famous "bullet" train from Kyoto to Tokyo. I was peacefully enjoying the greenness of the rice fields when suddenly there was a great commotion among the passengers. They all rushed to my side of the train to see an unusual sight. Thick creamy clouds had parted like a theater curtain, to reveal the incredible beauty and majesty of Mount Fuji.

The sight was soul-stirring. Picture postcards cannot convey the immensity of this mountain peak, nor its grandeur. Passengers exclaimed, quickly took pictures, and tried to record this beauty on their memories, for, true to form, in just a few minutes the clouds returned and hid Mount Fuji from our eyes.

That single incident changed the social climate in our car. People who had been strangers were chatting together. Others compared impressions of this gift of beauty that had touched us all and somehow united us as well.

Later, reflecting on that experience, I saw it as a symbol for each of us. After years of work as a counselor, I have come to the conclusion that the inner beauty of heart and soul in each person is most often hidden from view, like Mount Fuji. Clouds of self-doubt, guilt and fear keep this beauty hidden—not only from outsiders, but even from ourselves.

In my estimation, the work of a counselor or therapist is to help every client dispel these clouds, so that each person can experience his or her unique inner beauty and strength. The work of the counselor is not to attach labels to a person, nor to diagnose in order to prescribe. It is not, primarily, to give advice nor to solve problems. Clients are usually very good at the sort of self-analysis which ends in critical judgments and labeling. They do not need more reasons to feel guilty or ashamed. Instead, they need someone to help them unload the heavy burden of guilt and self-blame which they have been carrying by themselves.

I have discovered that clients who experience what Carl Rogers called "unconditional positive regard" also begin to experience greater inner resourcefulness. They stop seeking answers and magic solutions from the counselor and start examining ways to use their own inner power and creativity. This is so much better than applying the advice of an outside person. In the words of an ancient Zen proverb, they have been given not merely a fish; they have learned to fish for themselves. They have received not a mere panacea; they have been given a skill that lasts a lifetime.

Counselors who see their role in this way tend to focus on providing support and encouragement. They give their clients an environment that nurtures self-awareness. They aid them in uncovering their own inner beauty, and help them discover the ways in which they keep this inner grandeur hidden even from themselves. This process often awakens a sense of personal power which has long been dormant in the experience of the client.

The predominant feeling of a client who seeks out a counselor is one of powerlessness. It is the "I can't" experience. Developed over many years, sometimes from childhood, it leaves the person feeling helpless in the face of life's challenges. And very often this feeling of powerlessness stems from inner messages that have been believed: "You're no good," "You're too dumb," "You will never be a success." However, when the process is reversed; when the client begins to feel the faith of the counselor, he or she begins to feel some faith in himself or herself. The genuine acceptance of the counselor may trigger genuine acceptance of oneself. A gradual sense of personal power begins to grow as the client moves from the "I can't" experience to that of "Maybe I can...with a little help."

I see counseling as a relationship rather than a process of problem-solving. I *am* interested in the goal of our journey together, but I am more interested in what happens along the way. It is not techniques of counseling that attract me, but rather the development of a kind of loving presence between us. I am more concerned about the way *I am* with a person than in the things *I might do* with the person. I believe that it is the quality of this loving presence which enables a client to begin the move from powerlessness to a feeling of inner power.

I treasure the memory of a man who demonstrated this to me. He was an older Hawaiian with a gold tooth and a beautiful smile. I was nineteen years old and afraid of the water because of an unpleasant childhood experience in a swimming pool. I needed to learn to swim, and this man offered to teach me. He assured me that we would succeed, even though I remained doubtful. However, I accepted his offer and we went to a quiet little bay in Hawaii.

He looked into my eyes as we began the first lesson and said to me, "Do you trust me?" And though my inner fears were very loud, the love and caring in his eyes made me answer, "Yes." He then said, "Now, do just as I tell you, nothing more." And so we began a session in which I learned how to keep my face in water and turn it to get a breath. This was repeated for a couple of days. When I would ask, restless and impatient, "How soon do I learn to swim?" he would reply, flashing his gold tooth, "Bye-'n-bye."

Then it happened. One day he asked me to continue breathing and move my arms in a breast stroke until he told me to stop. I complied, and just when I was wondering if he had forgotten about me, he touched my hands and pulled me into shallow water. He asked me to stand and look back to the point from which I had begun my exercise.

It was a great distance away. He gave me a great hug and said, "Now, you can never again say 'I cannot swim,' because you just did!" It was a peak experience for me. I had moved from powerlessness to power, aided by the gentle, loving presence of this kindly Hawaiian. This gift also lasted a lifetime, for even today I swim far out to sea without fear. When I feel the water supporting me as I float on my back, I think of this man and utter a silent prayer of gratitude.

I believe that good counseling produces a similar experience, for similar reasons. Our feelings of powerlessness are usually the result of our fears. A strong, supportive presence enables us to let go of our fears, and activates our inner power. Love and fear seem to be opposite poles within us, controlling our feelings of power and our ability to release life-giving energy. If we are paralyzed by fear, we need to experience love in the form of caring, support and encouragement in order to counterbalance the effect of fear within us.

When I was new at counseling I put great emphasis on learning as many different approaches as possible. I attended workshops with most of the famous psychologists and therapists in the United States and Europe. I studied Gestalt and Primal Therapy, Bioenergetics and Art Therapy. I learned about yoga, Rolfing, body movement, Neo-Reichian therapy and hypnotism. I examined approaches using groups, from family therapy to encounter groups. I studied the ways of Zen Buddhism and transpersonal psychology, as well as journal writing and dream therapy.

Each of these ventures into work with other people gave me valuable new information. But the greatest value was a new awareness about myself. I discovered that the experiences which were the most effective for me were those which increased my sense of inner worth and personal power, and in which I could overcome my fears. Invariably this was associated with some person who communicated caring and acceptance of me, as well as a strong sense of inner assurance about himself or herself. I grew best with those people who were free from fear and thus free to create a loving presence for me.

So today, my emphasis is not on learning more techniques. My emphasis is on deepening my own sense of love, of restoring more quickly the balance I lose when I am afraid, and of consciously being aware of the need to create a loving presence for the client and myself.

Each day I spend a few moments in quiet reflection, a type of meditation, and when I am finished I usually discover that I have released some fear and anxiety. I have counterbalanced my negative thoughts with positive ones, and I have let go of some stress. As a result I feel new energy moving within, and feelings of loving gratitude arising in my heart.

I do a mini version of this balancing before each session with a client. I try to clear my mind of negative thoughts, relax my body from tension, and open my heart with love. It is then that I can offer a client what I call "the gift of a listening heart." This means that while I hear the verbalization of the client's problems, I am really listening to what he or she is feeling, to what the heart is saying. Usually it is a message rooted in some kind of fear. The words might be a woman's words of anger and resentment concerning her husband's behavior. But the heart may be saying, "I am afraid he no longer loves me."

When I am "balanced in love" it is then possible to create a relationship in which the client can begin to feel new worth and inner resourcefulness. My accepting both the expression of anger and the depth of the fear, and honoring these feelings, enables the energy which has been tied up in these negative emotions to be released. As our relationship strengthens, so do the client's feelings of personal power. Gradually, loving presence comes to be experienced in silence as well as through words, by a touch, or a look in the eyes, as well as through conversation.

As the client continues to grow, the mutuality of love seems to increase, so that the counseling process becomes more creative. There is greater permission and desire to share our time together in a lighter and more playful manner, rather than in the beginning, when everything seemed so serious and the problems so over-whelming. At this stage counseling may be a joy for both client and counselor, especially when the client discovers new alternatives and creative options where before there were only dead-end streets.

My effort today is directed toward achieving and maintaining this life-giving "love-balance." I am less concerned with "helping" the client than with sharing the loving presence that comes from inner balance. This means continuous work on my own personal growth rather than studying additional counseling approaches. It also means learning to be more sensitive to those things which trigger my own fears and areas of insecurity. Experience has shown me that only as I can dispel my own clouds of fear will I be able to join with my clients in dispelling theirs.

And that, ultimately, is what I seek. I want to create relationships with clients which make it possible for them to let go of these heavy burdens, to "push away the clouds" from their inner horizons so that they can experience their innate beauty and power. I believe this revelation will create a new life for them. They find, as did the passengers on the train who witnessed the beauty of Mount Fuji, that they begin to make new contacts with others. They are more open to risks and challenges. They are rewarded by other people, who respond to this sharing of themselves.

Rod McKuen has written a poem that speaks of these inner clouds, and of his need for a loving presence to help dispel them. I think it expresses well the experience of many of us. He writes:

If I had longer arms
I'd push the clouds away
or make them hang above the water somewhere else,

but...

I've never been able
to push the clouds away by myself.
Help me.

Please.

# CHAPTER TWO

# *The Gift of Heart-Listening*

It was early evening. The sun was casting long shadows against the flanks of the Koolau mountains, and cool winds hinted at a light rainfall. Even the bird-songs were gentle, reflecting the peace of sunset time in the Hawaiian countryside. I was visiting friends, and while they were getting ready to go out to dinner with me, I was enjoying a quiet meditation in their lovely garden.

Suddenly a car arrived at the outer gate, to the accompaniment of barking from the neighboring dogs. A man and woman with two young boys had arrived unexpectedly for a visit. They were greeted warmly by the couple. Introductions were made, and we all gathered together in the living room. My attention was drawn immediately to the youngest boy. He seemed hyperactive, jumping up and down in his chair, and making busy, repetitive movements with his hands. He did not speak, but instead made occasional low sounds. I promptly labeled him in my mind as "retarded" and began to covertly observe his behavior patterns.

Before long something took my attention away from the external behavior of the child, to an inner kind of reflection that touched me deeply. I became aware of the way in which my friends were responding to the visiting family and especially to this young boy. There was no sense of irritation at delayed dinner plans, only a feeling of warmth and enjoyment at being with people they cared about. I noticed the way in which they showed this caring differently to each member of the family—chatting, sharing experiences, playing and teasing. And even though I was not involved directly in most of these exchanges, I felt included somehow; touched by their tenderness and warmth.

Later, during dinner, we talked about the visit of this family. I realized that I had witnessed and been touched by a sharing in the expression of compassion—the special gift of a listening heart. That evening proved to be a rich learning experience for me. It stirred a great deal of reflection and gave birth to many new insights regarding this little-discussed expression of loving.

One of the insights concerns the difference between compassion and pity. David Brandon, in a marvelous little book called *Zen and the Art of Social Work*, points out that pity tends to dramatize the inferiority of the one receiving it. He defines pity as "one part sympathy and one part arrogance." Compassion, on the other hand, accepts and honors the one receiving it, because it comes from a heart pulsing in rhythm with that of the receiver. It is the gift of a heart that is attuned to the other person, able to hear and vibrate with the feelings of the other at a very deep level. Compassion tends to open doors rather than to close them. It is less concerned with finding answers than in offering support and examining possibilities. But most importantly,

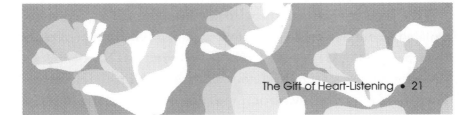

by being rooted in a listening with the heart rather than the rational, analytical mind, it enables us to transcend the usual quick critical judgments that so contaminate human relationships.

As I reflected on the way my friends responded to the visiting family, I realized that their compassionate response was the result of this beautiful heart-listening, which is rare in society today. I don't believe it is rare because people have closed their hearts to others. Many of us think we are being accepting and compassionate. It is not our intention to be critical. But the fact is that most of the time we listen with the head rather than the heart. There is something very challenging about solving mysteries, and when people tell us their problems we tend to focus on the external problems in an effort to solve them. We seek facts, examine circumstances, gather evidence, perhaps probe motivation, much in the manner of a detective trying to solve a murder case. Unfortunately our focus remains fixed at the level of the external problem.

It is only when we are able to listen with the heart that we are able to focus on the person as well as the problem. Then we are able to hear the powerful surge of inner fears, the warring forces of love and resentment, and perhaps the faint echo of buried hope. Our hearts tend to vibrate to these rhythms; we find ourselves "feeling with" the person. When expressed, these feelings offer the gift of compassion. This in turn touches the heart of the other person, who begins to feel understood and supported, not quite so alone, and a little less trapped. The touch of compassion brings to the receiver the feeling of companionship in the place of darkness; a dawning hope that with the help of this companion it might be possible to find a way out of the darkness.

The feeling of being supported rather than feeling alone and isolated is complemented by the experience of being accepted rather than being judged. A friend recalled the importance of this experience with respect to his father. He said, "During adolescence I knew my father was aware of my 'acting out,' especially in sexual behavior. I knew that my behavior ran counter to his moral and religious values. Yet he never criticized or scolded me in these matters. I felt his unspoken understanding very powerfully, and I knew he would be available if I needed him." This is an excellent example of the kind of heart-listening that finds expression in compassion.

A number of years ago I received a very important lesson that helped me to distinguish between what I thought was compassion and what was in reality a more self-centered desire to "help" someone less fortunate than me. I was counseling a man who was blind. At the end of one session I offered to accompany him across the street. I reached out, taking him by the arm, only to be stopped by him. He said to me, "Let me tell you how to help a blind person cross the street. First of all, don't take me by the arm. You are going to push me or pull me, and I may lose my balance. Also, I'll end up at the place *you* think I should be. Instead I would like you to offer me your arm. I will take as much or as little of your assistance as I need, and I will get safely to the place *I* want to be."

In the intervening years I have had many occasions to recall those words. During a counseling session when I may be thinking I am "helping" a person, the blind man's words sound in my mind like a bell ringing an alarm: "Don't push me or pull me...." And suddenly I realize that instead of listening to the client with love and compassion, I am subtly directing him or her towards the goal I think best. Invariably this awareness allows me to let go of my goal and become more of a compassionate companion for my client.

Sometimes listening with the heart not only enables me to hear a person more clearly, it also suggests an appropriate response. I

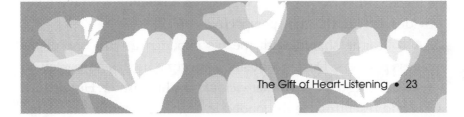

remember working with a woman who found it very difficult to talk about deep inner feelings. I sensed her need to not face me directly when she talked, and I suggested that we talk while walking along the beach. She found this helpful, and later I followed an intuitive prompting and asked her if she would like to help me plant some bulbs in my garden. I felt we could talk while we worked. She accepted my offer with a surprising amount of enthusiasm.

Each session thereafter we gardened together, and soon we had flowers to share. The work sessions in the garden provided the safe, warm atmosphere in which this woman could talk freely about her inner fears and conflicts without feeling criticized or judged by me. I discovered later that my invitation to garden enabled her to feel that *she* was helping *me,* and not merely taking the role of the person being helped. I sensed intuitively that this perspective was an essential prerequisite for her to establish an effective relationship with a counselor. She was touched not only by the appropriateness of the invitation, but also by the compassion that it represented.

Heart-listening and compassion are interwoven in such a marvelous way that they create a circle of caring. One gives rise to the other, and in turn is the result of the other. When we listen with the heart we begin to feel compassion in a new way, and when we feel compassion we also discover ourselves listening with the heart more spontaneously. This fact has special relevance to situations in which we are feeling anger or harboring resentment. During these times we tend to develop a fixed focus. We have evaluated the situation, assigned blame, and have focused fixedly upon being treated unfairly, or unjustly attacked. Our feelings cannot change unless we can see the situation from a new perspective. Listening with the heart provides us with this new perspective.

A colleague shared with me his experience with one of his business partners. During a business meeting my friend perceived himself as being attacked rather viciously by his partner. He felt hurt, angry and resentful. He responded in anger. The conflict escalated and brought the meeting to an abrupt ending. Later my friend spent time in meditation and found his heart speaking to him. He suddenly became aware that his partner had attacked him not because he wanted to hurt him, but because his partner had been afraid.

This new perspective changed his focus and his feelings. Anger and resentment gave way to compassion and understanding for a man who was under great stress from his marriage, a deteriorating physical condition, and financial difficulties. The next morning he called his partner, apologized for his angry remarks and invited him to lunch. The partner felt this genuine compassion and in turn shared some of the anguish behind his terrible feelings of insecurity. The meeting proved to be a healing session for both men. It illustrates the way in which heart-listening and compassion work together until they become responses that are readily available to us in any situation.

Compassion is not only a sensitive response to heart-listening; it can also be an expression of caring that is not afraid to be tough. There are times when we allow our fears to paralyze us, to keep us stuck, feeling helpless and impotent. Unlike the blind man, we need and want a little push to get started, to move off the stuck place. It is at such times that a compassionate person, hearing our silent heart-cry for help, can respond and help free us from our paralyzing fears.

Marilyn Ferguson, in the *The Aquarian Conspiracy*, quotes the poet Guillaume Appolinaire, who beautifully illustrates this aspect of compassion:

Come to the edge, he said.
They said: We are afraid.

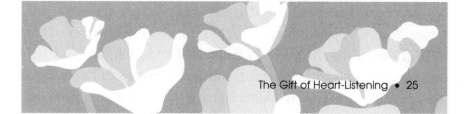

Come to the edge, he said.
They came.
He pushed them…and they flew.

Effective and satisfying life-changes occur only as a result of things that are deeply felt. The decisions that precede these changes require the strength and courage that compassion, born from heart-listening, can give us. The extra measure of loving energy enables us to listen with our hearts rather than our heads. Then we can make decisions based on what we know deep within us to be truly in our best interests. This gift is most often first experienced when given by a person who knows how to listen with the heart.

The Japanese have a special phrase to describe this kind of heart-listening. They speak of *kokorro-to-kokorro*, which means "heart speaking to heart." For them it is the most powerful form of communication because it is centered in love, and it is infallibly effective. They describe its effect as similar to a stone dropped into a clear pool. It sends out ripples in ever-widening circles, until the farthest reaches of the shore are touched by its gentle waves. Heart-listening sends out waves of love that wash away the waste of negative emotions and usher in a new energy of compassionate caring.

Heart-listening is rare mainly because we have not understood the importance of it. We thus do not take time to learn this beautiful and powerful art. Yet there seems to be a universal longing for this kind of communication. We want to be heard and understood by others at the deepest levels of our being. We want to be responded to with compassion. We all want to be in touch with the wisdom of our own hearts and be able to share this caring with others.

*Wanting to learn* this kind of listening is its essential prerequisite. By wanting, we open our hearts to the experience. It is not an art that is easily acquired. It demands discipline and attention and self-reflection, as well as the courage to take new risks. But the rewards are incredibly great for us and for those we touch with our listening.

The gift of heart-listening is, ultimately, the gift of our highest selves, and like all true gifts, one that enriches the giver as much as the receiver.

# CHAPTER THREE

## *The Lonely Pretense*

Recently I counseled a client who looked the picture of a successful career man. At thirty-five, with only a few gray streaks in his hair, he was a handsome and charming person who gave the impression of being in complete control of his life. However, just the opposite was true.

He had achieved many of his goals. He had a beautiful wife and family, and a business that had made him wealthy. He belonged to the right clubs and knew the right people. Externally, he gave the appearance of power and success, but within, he felt very frightened and very lonely. After several months of counseling he was able to release the cloud of fear that had overshadowed his life, and experience new inner power and confidence.

One of his most valuable insights was the realization that, from early childhood, he had learned that it was necessary to pretend. His well-meaning parents had trained him to deny and repress all negative feelings; to pretend to the world about him that "All is well and I am strong." He came to believe that being weak was a sin; an even greater sin was to allow other people to see this weakness.

As a result, this man became an accomplished actor. None of his childhood friends ever knew his real feelings or secret hurts. The pattern continued as an adult. Even his wife and children were strangers to his inner world. But throughout these long years he was in pain and unbearably lonely. Finally, in desperation, he sought counseling. There, for the first time in his life, he was able to say: "I am weak and needy, and I cannot bear this burden alone any longer."

Any counselor knows that this is not an unusual story. But what has surprised me as I reflect on my experiences with people, old and young, is just how common it is. In fact, this pattern seems to be true for most of us. We all learn in early childhood that our culture rewards strength and punishes weakness. Most of us discover very soon that winning is the great goal, and losing is the great shame; that succeeding is what matters and failing is inexcusable. And so our fears begin to grow: fear of not being good enough; fear of being weak; fear of being needy, fear of failing. Above all is the fear of letting anyone know about our inner pain.

I clearly recall my own first experience of mistrust. When I was four years old, my family moved to a new area. One of my first outings was to a birthday party. I enjoyed the games, even though most of the children were strangers to me. On leaving, we were all given popcorn balls as a gift. Then we piled into a pick-up truck to be taken home. Suddenly, I remembered I had left my sweater in the house. I asked the driver to wait, told my companions to hold my popcorn ball for me, and ran back to get my sweater. When I returned, the other children were eating my popcorn ball and laughing at me.

I was stunned. I had never experienced a similar misplacement of trust, and their action seemed very cruel. But even at that tender age I knew how to react. Despite my aching heart, I laughed at those children and said to them, "Hah! The joke's on you. I don't like popcorn balls, so eat it all up!" By age four I had already learned that the worst sin is to let someone discover your hidden hurt.

I wonder how many of us are still operating by this principle? We keep our inner worlds very private. Most of us try to carry our burdens alone, pulling ourselves up by our own bootstraps. We read the famous line of Saint Paul, exhorting us to "bear the burdens of one another," and we interpret that to mean that we must help others only, and not that others are to help us. If we have this outlook, we need to re-examine some of our childhood beliefs and assumptions.

First, we need to create a balance between "doing it myself" and "letting others help me," between rugged individualism and de-pendent leeching. Keeping my inner world as an absolutely inviolable sanctuary is as crazy as allowing everyone to know everything about me. Both are extremes. I do need a part of myself, and perhaps some of my history, to be considered my private possession. But I also need to share some of my inner feelings with one or more trusted people. I need this if only to gain a realistic perspective, for that is what we usually lose when we enter our private worlds alone. The mind conjures up countless fears, which cast shadows over reality and lead us to false conclusions.

A loving friend who knows how to listen rather than advise can help us find a perspective which restores the balance of reality. We can come to see, perhaps, that our demands on ourselves have been unrealistic. We discover that being human means that sometimes we are strong and sometimes weak; that sometimes we succeed and sometimes fail, and that both can yield important life-experiences. For example, in sports it is extremely important for a young person to learn how to lose. Learning to be a gracious winner is useful, but as a life-lesson it is even more important that we learn how to be a humble and creative loser.

I remember seeing a film of a remarkable psychiatrist who was training mentally retarded men and women to assemble a bicycle brake. When they would fail to assemble one part correctly, he would simply say to them, very gently, "Try another way." The trainee would then reverse the part, and discover that it fit perfectly. These young people not only learned to assemble the brakes efficiently, they acquired a motto to help them with apparent failure: *Try another way*. I think this motto could benefit all of us when we are inclined to analyze our failures rather than trying new, creative alternatives.

Many people receiving counseling make this mistake. After clients describe their experiences with failure, they proceed to analyze them. Sometimes this is necessary; but my preference is to help them to search out new possibilities, to trigger their latent personal power. Then, *after* the person begins to feel new energy and new hope, we might go back to the situation that produced the failure. Sometimes this is not needed. For some fortunate people, the desire to create a new experience is greater than the need to dwell on a past mistake.

Many people are reluctant to surrender their urge to re-examine. A particular woman who came to me for counseling seemed to hold tenaciously on to this desire for self-dissection. Only through humor and a loving teasing did she come to see herself like a dog with a bone—refusing to let go even when it served no positive purpose. She finally came to realize that her obsessive analysis usually led to self-scolding and depression.

This is almost universally true. Focusing on past failure rarely, if ever, gives us new energy. Instead it drains us of energy by re-awakening old fears. A famous story tells of a disciple of Buddha who was in the habit of analyzing past situations. The Buddha is said to have told him this story:

"Imagine that a soldier has been wounded with a poisoned arrow. The doctor arrives to remove the arrow, but before he can do anything the soldier says, 'Wait! Before you take out the arrow, I want some information. I want to know who shot the arrow, why he shot it, what he looks like,' and so on. Now if the doctor stops to answer all the questions, what do you think will happen to the soldier?"

The disciple said, "He will most likely die."

The Buddha replied, "It is the same with your questions. I have no intention of being concerned about your speculation and analyzing. I am interested only in teaching you how to put an end to suffering."

We must resist the temptation to merely focus on an examination of the past. We need, instead, to do something to alter our present perspective.

In addition to changing our perspective of failure, it is also necessary, for many of us, to change our perspective of success. A surprisingly large number of externally "successful" men are actually terrified of their success. Like the businessman who had learned to mask his feelings, they have become good actors who live constantly under the shadow of many fears. They are afraid of the constant challenge to remain successful; they fear change of any kind; they fear the threat of their multiple responsibilities, and they fear the uncertainty of the future. In addition, many of the negative messages from childhood rise from the past to haunt them. And because they cannot share these terrible fears with anyone, they carry them alone and suffer tragic loneliness. Some turn to alcohol or drugs. Others develop ulcers or heart attacks from the stress. And a few seek counseling.

Their stories are remarkably similar. From childhood they felt torn and confused by parental demands to succeed, mixed with accusations that they were either incompetent or unlikely to succeed. Their need for parental approval became a motivating force, and they determined to win their parents' love. But inside, many of these men felt it was all a charade. They felt unworthy of their own success, believing that it comes more through fate than their ability. The lives of many of these men demonstrate the Peter Principle. They were frequently more secure and happier when in less responsible, less successful positions. Some made excellent workers and poor managers.

In a fair number of these cases, the "Peter Pan Syndrome" is also at work. These are men, as described by Dr. Dan Kiley in his book of the same name, who never want to grow up. They want to remain little boys; they fear adult responsibilities. They become very creative at escaping efforts to turn them into responsible adults. They drop out of school, they get fired from jobs, they develop mysterious and exotic illnesses. And yet, because many of them are charming, they are able to become successful in business by getting others to assume many of their responsibilities. But all the while they are frightened and unhappy with their success.

The fear of success is certainly not limited to men. It is appearing in growing numbers of young women who are moving up the career ladder. They have learned to compete effectively with men, but they have not learned to be comfortable with success. Colette Dowling, in her book *The Cinderella Complex*, describes her own battle with these fears as she tried to juggle a second marriage with a career, and found herself sabotaging possible success as a writer.

The stress is especially heavy for young women who feel that they must not only be as good as men, but must be better than men if they are to reach the top. And even though women in general are more willing to share their inner selves with others, these career women seem to feel that they must keep their secret fears to themselves. So like the men with whom they compete, they show a good front to the world, and carry their secret burden alone.

The only path that takes both men and women out of the dark forests of fear and pretense is the path of sharing their burdens with others. In his famous work *The Divine Comedy*, Dante describes the beginning of a journey which takes him through hell and into heaven. It starts at the edge of a dark and frightening wooded place, and Dante is terrified at the prospect of entering this place. But he feels somewhat more confident when Virgil appears and offers to be his companion and guide.

Together they enter the forest, confront the shadows and spirits, and ultimately arrive at a place of light and exquisite beauty. For Dante, the beauty of heaven is only part of his discovery. The other reward is the realization that a person does not have to wait for heaven in order to find life's meaning. When one has a loving companion, *the journey itself has meaning and purpose.* It gives support and enrichment, and enables us to abandon our fears. Together we can face the darkness, and feel secure that our combined strength will overcome the obstacles we meet.

For me, one of the greatest gifts that a loving friend can offer is acceptance. When someone knows us intimately, we no longer have to pretend. We can abandon not only some of our fears, but also our need to always put up a good front. This makes our journey a much freer and lighter experience. This is one of the experiences that people who seek counseling value highly: being with a trusted friend who knows and loves them, warts and all. It is like coming into a cozy living room with a roaring fire, after a long walk in a winter storm.

It seems strange that the spirit of rugged individualism, which helped build America into a powerful nation, should become the source of so much personal pain. But it is true. We have carried the concept to an extreme which is inhuman. It has made us feel that we must achieve success, solve our problems, overcome our obstacles and bear our burdens, all by ourselves. This is an impossible dream. It separates us from the very people who could help us accomplish all of these things, and it leaves us terribly lonely.

I recall a middle-aged woman in an encounter group who shared some of her secret inner fears, admitting that this was the first time she had ever disclosed such weakness. After she shared these things, with a few tears, I reached out, and, touching her arm, said very simply, "Welcome to the human race." My remark was not very original, but it was sincere. Some time later she wrote me a letter in which she said that those few words struck a chord deep within her, adding, "I now realize that being weak is nothing more than being me at that moment, and it's okay. Besides, it feels so good not to have to be Superwoman for everyone anymore. Those days are gone. I also notice that people are much warmer than before and it feels very good to me."

This woman's experience dramatizes the liberating effects of sharing our humanness with others. Sharing our weakness, our burdens, our fears, with trusted and caring people brings us not only greater personal strength, but a sense of togetherness that can turn a frightening journey into an exciting adventure.

Barbara Streisand's hit song from *Funny Girl* says it well: "People who need people are the luckiest people in the world."

CHAPTER FOUR

# *The Other Side of Caring*

Recently I read a newspaper account of a young man who had left teaching to become a salesman. Yet two years previously he was honored by his state as "Teacher of the Year." People wondered, "How come? What happened?" An interview revealed his reasons for leaving the teaching profession.

"I was burnt-out. Classes were too large. The one-on-one contact with my students, which was most satisfying for me, was very limited. I spent most of my time doing reports and attending endless faculty meetings which accomplished little. Finally I said, "I've had it." This work is too frustrating and unfulfilling for me. I need a career that offers greater emotional and financial rewards."

This teacher's decision is not unique. Men and women in the caring professions are leaving for similar reasons. Nurses are accepting jobs in research or consulting, social workers are switching to brokerage houses. A woman I know left her job as a counselor for battered women to become an office manager for an advertising firm.

These choices reveal not only the heavy burden of jobs in the caring professions. They also dramatize what might be termed *the other side of caring*.

Usually we think of caring as an expression of love. But the coin of caring has another side. Caring can be self-centered as well as other-centered. Without realizing it, we may be feeding others primarily in order that we might be fed. I am not suggesting that this was so in the case of the young teacher; I identify closely with his experience, being a teacher myself. But I also know that much of my own pain has been the result of the darker side of my caring, and his dilemma has prompted me to examine this aspect a little more closely.

Sometimes the language we use to express caring gives us away. We smile at parents who say to their children, as they are administering punishment, "It's only because I care." We smile because we know that the remark is a half-truth at best. We are annoyed when well-intentioned friends give us advice, adding, "I wouldn't say this if I didn't care." If the advice is unsolicited, as it often is, we are inclined to say to ourselves, "Who asked you?" If the advice is poor advice, as also happens frequently, we might ask, "With friends caring like this, who needs enemies?"

The point is that underneath our words of caring is behavior which reveals more self-interest than genuine concern for others' needs. And while it is true that caring will always contain a certain mixture of self-centered love and other-centered love, our problems usually arise from the *degree* of self-love and from *our lack of awareness of that degree*. Most of our pain comes from the "too-much" quality of our caring.

We are all familiar with the "Jewish mother syndrome." The label

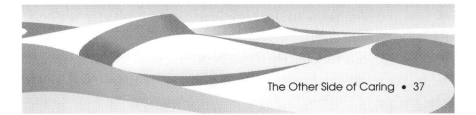

is unfair and racist, since Irish, Italian, African and Asian mothers all act this way. And not only mothers are the culprits, but fathers, teachers, lovers and therapists. The reality behind the label is one of caring too much. Such people want the very best for those they love, expressing their love in phrases like: "Nothing is too good for my child"; "I want him or her to have all the things I didn't have as a child." These people are generous and make great sacrifices, but it is often "in order that." Whatever qualifications follow indicate the carers' hopes, dreams and expectations for the loved ones. They are unaware that their caring may be self-centered and suffocating.

When I was a novice counselor, my supervisor helped me to realize how much my own self-interest was involved in my work with clients. Reviewing a particular session, this man asked, very gently, "When you asked that question of the client, whose needs do you think you were meeting?" I did not like the question, nor the answer it uncovered: "My own." A gesture that I thought was helping the client actually revealed my own need to be reassured that I was a competent and caring counselor.

This need for approval subtly tempts us down a dead-end road of too much caring. We give a great deal to others so that we will be told in words and by actions that we are lovable, understanding, nice people. But it creates terrible conflicts for us.

I see this so often with student teachers. They love the challenge of teaching and the reward of seeing students learn. But the combination of their too-much caring and their need to be liked causes untold pain for them when they must grade the students. They want so badly for "their children" to do well, and they do not want to be seen as meanies. They frequently fail to see that genuine caring respects and honors the student's right to have whatever grade he or she has chosen to earn.

*Failing to see* is the effect of the distortion caused by our too-much caring. We imply this by our use of the phrase, "Love is blind." Fritz Perls, father of Gestalt Therapy, added another dimension to this insight. He believed a common problem in relationships arose from our perception of "falling in love." We think we are falling in love with a person, whereas we often are falling in love *with our image of what that person can become*. When the person fails to live up to our image we are unhappy and angry.

When too-caring parents are confronted with the destructive or criminal behavior of their children, their common reaction is: "My child would never do such things!" It is hard to let go of the image and accept the person *as is*.

How then do we find our way out of the maze of problems created by our caring? Strange as it may seem, our disappointment can be the first step to freedom. Disappointment can be an inner alarm clock telling us it is time to wake up. The sadness we feel can be a message informing us that our too-much caring has taken over. A colleague of mine tells how this happened in his own life. He says, "I was so excited with the progress of one of my clients that I became like a cheerleader for him. I encouraged him to move faster and rewarded him with my approval. I was devastated when he did not come to see me for over a month.

"And then the bell rang! I could see by my disappointment how much my own needs were involved in his growth. This insight was confirmed when finally he did return and said to me, 'You were pushing me too hard. I couldn't live up to your expectations. And when I fell off the pedestal you put me on I was too ashamed to come back.' What a lesson for me! It was humbling but valuable."

Facing and feeling our disappointment can be like following a beacon of light which guides us out of the maze of our confusion. With added light we are able to confront the darker side of our caring and see *what is* rather than *what might be*.

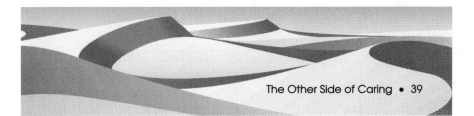

Our too-much caring is neither needed nor wanted by the people we love. Our supposed gift of love is a burden of dependency for both people. What we are certain is unconditional love is frequently conditional love which says, "I will love you if you behave as I think you should. If you don't, I will be hurt and disappointed." A clearer vision of reality enables us to appreciate the darker side of caring. Through it, we can develop into genuinely loving persons.

With brighter light and new insights, we come to the final quality that gives us the energy to move out of the maze, and this is humor. We even begin to laugh at our too-much caring. A friend of mine does this so well. This warm, generous woman occasionally finds herself back in the old familiar pattern of too-much caring. And when she hears the alarm of her disappointment ringing, she laughs and says, "Damn, damn, damn! I did it again! Well, that's that! Now I can start *really* loving that person."

When we can respond like this, we are able to switch the focus back to caring for another person in a way that is freeing and nurturing for both of us. The essence of this focus is beautifully expressed in the prayer attributed to Saint Francis:

O Divine Master, grant that I may not so much seek
To be consoled, as to console
To be understood, as to understand
To be loved, as to love...

It is this focus which keeps in balance the brighter and darker sides of our caring.

CHAPTER FIVE

# *Creative Giving*

In recent years I have spent extended periods of time in Japan. Each time I return home from one of these trips I am laden with gifts from friends and clients. And although I am warmed by their generosity, I am most touched by the sensitivity and creativity of their gift-giving. Let me give an example.

During one of my first workshops in Japan I formed a friendship with a training manager of a large Japanese corporation. I shared with this man my love for Hawaii, with its clear blue skies and sea the color of pale jade. He said he would like very much to visit Hawaii and experience that beauty first-hand. As I was departing from the airport, my friend came to the terminal with a gift. It was a small, rough ceramic tea cup which he had had one of his friends make especially for me. Around the rim of the cup was a glaze the color of pale jade.

I was deeply touched by the gift, for it said so much more than words could ever have expressed. Besides the sheer beauty of the cup, the message it conveyed was: "When you drink from this cup, think of me until we can drink tea together by the sea that is the color of pale jade."

The teacup was an expression of creative giving. The gift becomes more than an object of beauty. It becomes a link between friends, a connection of two hearts. It contains memories of the past as well as a bridge to future sharings. In addition, this particular gift awakened in me the value and power of creative giving. I realize that while this kind of giving is almost second nature for the Japanese, it is an art that many of us in the West have yet to learn. Fortunately, many of us have been blessed with one or two people in our lives who have acquired this art: the person who can select the perfect card for some special occasion, or the one person who finds an unusual gift to touch our hearts. Yet even with these models in our lives, most of us need to reflect upon the aspects of their giving that make it so special and creative.

I recall a woman who had a great impact on my own life. She was a warm, exuberant person whose love for life was matched only by her generosity. Through her I came to an understanding and appreciation of opera, ballet and classical music. Sensing my need to grow musically, she invited me to join her party attending some concerts. She explained, simply, the structure of a symphony or concerto. Several times she invited me backstage to meet some of the musical celebrities whom she knew. It was heady stuff for an adolescent, and I loved it.

Only later did I discover that this kind of sensitive caring toward me was characteristic of this woman in her relationships with many people. She had a marvelous ability to tune in to a person's needs and to find a delicate way to respond to those needs. To one person she would give an expensive gift, to another, a gift she had made with her own hands. On one occasion she gave a wonderful gift to an actor who was out of work. She gave him a surprise party, arriving with friends she had collected and food she had prepared. Her giving had a way of sharing her joy in life and of warming the heart of the receiver, so that acceptance was a delight rather than a burden of embarrassment. I have found this to be a characteristic of most creative givers I have known.

Another quality that seems to distinguish creative givers is the ready willingness to share *themselves* as well as material possessions. They give freely and generously of their time and energy. They offer their compassion and caring spontaneously, as it is needed by others. These people are, for me, modern counterparts of the biblical Good Samaritan, who was willing to walk the extra mile, put aside his own cares and needs, in order to bind up the wounds of someone else. This generous, and at times even lavish, gift of self, has a powerful impact upon a person who needs loving support and inner healing.

Eastern writers enjoy drawing our attention to this quality in nature. They remind us that apple trees do not cling to their blossoms. Rather, they share this beauty lavishly in springtime, and in summer they freely offer the gift of their fruit to all who desire it. This is especially clear to anyone who has visited a tropical or semi-tropical region. Living in Hawaii, I am constantly reminded of the lavish generosity of nature: lovely rain forests and valleys alive with the many-splendored hues of green: plumeria, ginger and pikake fragrances filling whole areas with their lush, sweet scent; mangoes and papaya so abundant that in early summer people have difficulty giving away their rich harvests.

Nature's generous and universal sharing can serve as a model and reminder for us of another way of being: a more creative way of living through a more creative approach to giving. We need such reminders when we find ourselves stuck in a pattern of self-interest and attachment, of believing that by holding on to things we can really keep them for ourselves. Nature teaches us an alternate way. By letting go, we are able to experience new growth; by emptying out, we free ourselves to be filled anew; in the process of giving lavishly, we find ourselves enriched.

Several years ago I was attending a staff meeting with a remarkable group of people who had formed a close-knit community. During the meeting, one of the senior staff members was sharing some personal anguish resulting from a painful disappointment. A number of staff members offered gifts of understanding and support, but one person offered a most sensitive and valued gift. Grasping the hand of the senior member, this woman said, "I am keenly aware of your pain and also your courage in having kept this to yourself, but right now, for all of us who love you, I would like to give you permission to cry." And with a great sigh of relief, the man slowly let the tears fall, saying later, "Thanks so much for that gift. I really needed that permission."

This incident led me to reflect upon similar needs that we all have, needs that could be satisfied by other forms of creative giving: the gift of silent presence when the hurt is too great to discuss; the gift of a loving touch that offers only affection and compassion without any demands. Such creative gifts follow our tuning in to the hidden, inner, real needs of people. These gifts come from the heart and touch the hearts of those who receive them.

Creative givers have another quality I admire. They are not only generous and even lavish in giving; they are gracious in receiving

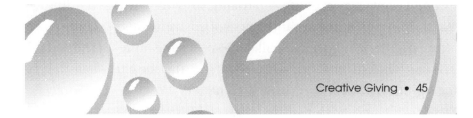

gifts. This quality in itself can be a form of creative giving. One of the most loving things we can do for a person who offers us a gift is to accept it with love and gratitude.

Like many professional helpers, I have been much better at giving to others than in allowing others to give to me. But I have been fortunate through the years in having good models, people who have shown me how to receive gifts lovingly, whether these be words of praise and appreciation, or material gifts. I learned that my reluctance to receive these gifts was really an expression of my inner fears; it was also dishonest. Although I was usually touched by the caring, I was embarrassed by a public expression of it and felt a bit out of control. I was, in effect, rejecting both the gift and the love behind the gift, because of my own insecurity. I began to try to act differently. I found that it was not difficult to say "Thank you" with genuine love and gratitude. As a result I began to feel good, not only about the gift and the giver, but also about myself and my ability to return love with love.

Creative giving seems to liberate us from our tight, narrow little worlds. It widens our horizons, softens our critical judgments and deepens our compassion. As we change our focus from getting to giving, wonderful things begin to happen. People who practice tithing give eloquent testimony to significant transformations in their lives once their attitudes towards giving and receiving began to change.

Creative giving liberates each of us in a different way, obviously. But the form of the liberation is not as important as the fact of the liberation, for freedom in any area of life tends to grow and diffuse through every aspect of life. Gradually, as we come to better understand the symbolic nature and power of giving, we also become more attuned to the symbols that will have special meaning for individual persons. The gift itself becomes secondary. It is the *gift behind the gift*, the significance of this gesture, that matters. We come to appreciate the attitude and advice of the medieval writer Thomas à Kempis, who said, "Think not so much of the gift of the lover, as the love of the giver." In this mindset, a phone call, a special card, a single flower, the touch of a hand, a souvenir, a funny story, a silent walking companion, can be gifts that though small in themselves are great in their loving impact.

At its best, creative giving brings the divine into the most ordinary moment. It brings a touch of love that is eternal, universal, lavish and compassionate. It re-creates both the giver and the receiver, and replicates itself in further acts of giving.

Creative giving is a kind of "lovestone" dropped into the pond of human life. We can touch even the most distant shore by a single generous gift of self. When the giver looks into the rippled pond he or she is doubly enchanted by the beauty seen: first, by the perfection of the expanding concentric circles, and as the waters become calm, by the divine beauty of his or her own reflection.

This is the ultimate gift of creative love.

# CHAPTER SIX

# Seed-Planting and Harvesting

In the age of instant coffee, satellite communication and television replays, we have become accustomed to immediate responses. Despite the obvious advantages of this kind of efficiency, there are some drawbacks. One of these is a lessening of our appreciation for things that do not happen immediately. By focusing so much on immediate results, we tend to identify results solely with the visible response or lack of it. In other words, whenever we do not get an immediate reaction or when we cannot see an immediate result, we are tempted to think that nothing is going to result. This habit confuses *seed planting* with *harvesting*.

Some things do indeed furnish us with an instant response; others, like seeds, make us wait for a while before they give evidence of the good work that has already taken place.

For many years of my life I was addicted to harvesting. I did not want to put energy into situations or people from which I could not derive some immediate satisfaction. I chose a career in sales as opposed to teaching for this reason. Later, I found rewards in lecturing because you get an immediate response from your audience. They are either with you or against you, and the sound of enthusiastic applause confirms the success of your efforts. Throughout this early part of my career I seemed to need the security of this immediate response.

Then I began my life-work as a counselor. I listened to people in pain and confusion, describing their problems and fears, seeking a way out of the myriad mazes of their dilemmas. I worked with them, walked beside them, cared for them, supported them. I was able to help many of them change their poor self-images and begin to activate their own inner resources. These people gave me some immediate response. I could see them changing and growing, and I felt rewarded, knowing that, in some small way, I was a part of that growth process.

But there were others who were a source of disappointment for me, people who seemed to remain stuck in their tragic life scripts; people who appeared to be unable, unwilling or too afraid to take the risks that would produce new growth. I could not see any positive effects emerging from my work with them, and I judged myself a failure because of this. I felt guilty, wondering what else I might have done to help them. I realize now that I was not thinking about seed planting at all. I was focusing on harvesting, and because I saw no sign of the harvest, I assumed that no seeds had been planted.

My awakening came one day when I received a call from one of these "unharvested" clients and was invited to lunch. During the meal I listened with astonishment to a recital of incredible personal growth during the year that had intervened since our last session.

Gone were the old fears and self-doubts that had imprisoned this woman. Gone was the desperate clinging to others for approval. Instead she radiated self-assurance and inner strength. She had ended a disastrous relationship and was beginning one which was more supportive for her. She had quit her old job and gone into business for herself. She was struggling, but loving the challenge, and certain that she would make a success of it. I could scarcely believe the words I was hearing, but the poised, confident woman sitting across the table from me—completely transformed from her former self—dispelled any lingering doubts about the new reality she was describing.

One of the most pleasant surprises for me was her reference to a number of our counseling sessions. She recalled things I had said, role-playing we had done, times when I was able to tease her out of her self-pity. Bit by bit, these insights fell into place to form a lovely mosaic of growth within her. It took time and patience in order for this integration to occur. Seeds had been planted, but the growth needed slow nurturing before the harvest could be seen.

That luncheon meeting stimulated some new growth in me. I became aware that the really important work in counseling is seed planting, not harvesting. As a result I began to change my focus. Today I am interested in helping a client to plant seeds; I do not need to see immediate signs of growth. Since changing my focus, I have become aware that some of the best growth occurs after the counseling sessions, not during them. I am content to put my energy into the way I am with the client, rather than looking for immediate results.

Over the years the appropriateness of my change in focus has been validated may times. A number of clients have told me, either in person or by letter, that a particular interaction in a previous counseling session had had great significance for them. It prompted a genuine "Aha!" for them—yet I had no awareness of this fact at the time. Seeds had been planted, and growth begun, without my knowledge. I experienced a similar change during my work with encounter groups. In the past I had made judgments about the worth of these groups. I would say, "This one was a success; that one a failure," or "This group was dull, and nothing much happened."

I no longer make these judgments. Too many people have given me feedback like, "That group changed my life" or "That group enabled me to feel good about myself for the first time in my life," long after a group experience which I may have labeled "dull" or "a failure." Today I am less inclined to make value judgments about group experiences. I am more satisfied to believe that, very likely, seeds have been planted, and growth will occur in due time.

Focusing on seed planting as opposed to harvesting is difficult for young counselors. I see most student counselors struggling with this situation; for some it can be a great handicap to their effectiveness. Their need to see results can prompt them to push their clients towards growth for which the clients are not ready. At other times, this need for results can obscure the reality of growth already begun but not yet manifested. Sometimes it takes a dramatic experience for these students to change their focus, to be aware of their own distortion.

On one occasion, in a counseling class, I was demonstrating the use of Gestalt in dream work. I chose a student who felt that a recent dream had hidden meaning for him. At the beginning of the demonstration I explained my method of working and asked the class to withhold judgment as to the effectiveness of the method based on observable effects. I wanted them to concentrate on the process rather than the results.

The session lasted perhaps fifteen minutes. The student followed my directions in acting out parts of the dream, but it was apparent that he was struggling with himself and, at times, resisting the process. At one point he came close to tears and quickly suppressed them. When the session was over I could sense the disappointment of the students who had been observing. I could imagine them saying to themselves, "I don't think the Gestalt approach is very effective; nothing much happened." For my part I felt good about the session and believed that some significant seeds had taken root.

The following day that same student came to me and said, "A fantastic thing happened to me after class yesterday. I got home and was unusually restless. I tried a number of diversions but I just could not relax. Finally I realized what was bothering me. In my work on the dream I became aware of part of the cause of my poor relationship with my father, and I had a powerful need to talk to him. I went over to see him and was able to do what I had wanted to do for years. I told him that I loved him and that I knew he loved me. I also said that I realized my mistake in insisting that he love me my way, when it was not possible for him to do this. I added that I am now able to let him love me his way and be grateful for that love.

"I saw my father's eyes fill with tears, and we embraced for the first time as grown men. It was a wonderful, healing experience for us both. And it was a direct result of the things that got stirred up in me during our dream session in class. I want to share this story with the whole class so they can appreciate how much took place that was not apparent yesterday afternoon."

It is vitally important that we receive encouragement for our planting of these hidden seeds, because there are many times we find our patience growing thin, especially after repeated efforts to help people. One of the greatest sources of encouragement for me has been the discovery of what happens when we actually do walk the extra mile.

A number of times I have been tempted to give up on certain clients. Nothing I could say or do seemed to help these people. They appeared to be trapped, powerless, hopeless. All my caring efforts seemed like seeds falling on sterile soil. Yet something in me would not give up. I continued to treat these people with love and caring. Some I would call and say "Hello" or wish them well; to others I would send a note or card to reassure them that I cared and was thinking of them. And from many of these clients I received warm and touching letters, perhaps telling me that my note reached them when they were lonely and even desperate. The sense that I was somehow with them enabled a number of people to activate their own inner forces and make changes, or ask others for help. These incidents awaken me again and again to the hidden power in acts of caring which plant and nurture the seeds of change.

Our need to see results, to enjoy the harvesting, is somewhat like our attitude toward gift-giving. We see another person confused or frightened and want to offer support and reassurance. It is our intention to genuinely and generously offer a gift to someone in need. But our own need to see results, to know that our gift of love is accepted and appreciated, often reveals more self-concern than true love.

Gift-giving means simply giving a gift to another person without any strings or conditions. There is no demand for acknowledgment or expressions of gratitude. When we give a gift of love with these demands, we are involved in a form of extortion: "I will give you a gift on the condition that you pay me in gratitude." Swami Satchidananda, an Indian yogi, says that this type of giving is less like an act of love and more like a business transaction. Most recipients sense this hidden demand and resent it.

When I was a child, my grandmother had a wonderful way of dealing with this type of giving. She gave away the gifts that were given to her. The family was well aware of Grandma's predisposition. We would see our Christmas gifts being shared with friends or other relatives on birthdays and celebrations, and we did not like it.

So, when the next occasion appeared for giving gifts to Grandma we would pointedly say, "Now, Grandma, this is for *you*, so use it and enjoy it, and don't give it away." Grandmother would smile her sweetest smile and say, "Why thank you, what a nice gift." Then she would add, "And you did say you were giving this to me, didn't you?"

After our assurances that this was indeed true, Grandma would utter the final crushing statement: "Then if you are giving it to me, it is mine, and I can then dispose of it as I please. Thank you again for the gift." We never got the better of Grandma in these exchanges. She continued to use some of our gifts and make presents of the rest of them. The lesson was clear: "Don't give me a gift if there are any conditions attached to it, because then it really isn't a gift."

When we are centered in love, we can give from the heart and not need to see results in the form of expressions of appreciation. When we are centered in love we are content with seed-planting rather than needing to reap the harvest. Then in working with people, in helping others, our seed-planting becomes genuine gift-giving. The powerful chemistry of love is able to stimulate growth. Seeds then get continual nourishment, growing into sturdy plants that, in turn, nourish others. People grow to love themselves and share this love with others.

Finally, this love-sharing comes back to the original seed planter in many mysterious ways, and the circle is complete. Until this happens, we can stay more centered in love by focusing on unconditional gift-giving. At the same time, we enjoy more inner peace and satisfaction, knowing that in a small way, we have done something truly wonderful. In love, we have planted the seeds of new life.

CHAPTER SEVEN

# *Caring for the Caretakers*

It was an early evening appointment. The afterglow from the setting sun filled my office with a soft light. Cool ocean breezes caused the venetian blinds to swing gently against the window. The tranquil scene was a dramatic contrast to the outpouring of anguish from the man seated opposite me. He gave the appearance of a young man who was successful, in control of his life. Yet he had just finished describing his marriage at a battleground, his health as marginal, and his inner resources as depleted. He was a social worker, a caretaker of others, who had forgotten the importance of caring for himself. The work that had been rewarding had become a heavy burden. He said, "Sometimes I would love to just hop in my car and get away from it all, but I would feel guilty about abandoning my clients. So I hang in there and try to help them, but I'm not even doing a very good job at that any more."

The social worker was experiencing what is currently called "burn-out." The term describes people who are physically over-worked and emotionally undernourished. A psychologist expressed his feeling this way, "It seems as if all my energy is going out to others and nothing is coming back, and I don't know how to change this." I have heard similar statements from doctors, nurses, psychologists and educators, people involved in helping professions. The effects upon their lives can be seen in troubled love relationships, escapes into drugs or alcohol, along with increasing feelings of isolation and impotence. The courage of adults gives way to the fear and insecurity of children. The present is unbearable and the future appears bleak.

In seeking ways to help them replace these negative experiences with more positive ones, I have come to some insights about the art of self-care for professionals.

Healing professionals tend to see themselves as gifted, skilled and trained in the art of caring for others. We feel good about these qualities, and confident in our ability to help others. Yet many of us do not feel adequately trained in caring for ourselves. When we find our energy low, our spirits depressed, and the burdens of our profession heavy, we do not feel able to utilize the resources within us to alter our own negative emotions. Professional helpers urgently need a practical education in the delicate and important art of caring for ourselves.

Most find it difficult to ask for help, and even more difficult to accept help when offered. Caretakers are good at giving and rather poor at receiving. So the art of receiving is an important part of our professional and personal re-education.

I also discovered that many professional clients have lost contact with their bodies and with the world of nature. When their energy is low, they tend to play harder, or to eat and drink more than is good for them. They are not open to nature, and thus do not experience its relaxing and nourishing effects. It is necessary to educate them anew in the art of sensitive listening to their bodies and to nature.

Perhaps the most significant learning is the realization of how much all professionals need to recognize our own negative patterns of thinking. These patterns reinforce our feelings of powerlessness and helplessness. We need help to become aware of such thinking and find ways to correct the imbalance.

A caring relationship is vital for professional caretakers. In counseling them I have found that the things we *said* were not nearly as significant as the things we *did* and *shared* together. Gradually a caring relationship began to be built, and in this environment, the re-education process could flourish. New insights and new choices, new ways of seeing reality and new kinds of behavior began to appear. New feelings of inner worth and self-confidence came to replace the hopeless/helpless attitudes that had paralyzed some of these men and women.

It was apparent from the beginning that just talking about the problems would not be adequate for these caretakers. Their basic concern was on the emotional rather than on the intellectual level. They needed an *experience* of caring, rather than a *verbal discussion about* caring. Although this is true for all clients, it is especially needed by professionals. One of the advantages in working with professionals is their high degree of motivation. They are hurting and they want to feel alive and well again. They also place a great deal of trust in me; this makes it possible for me to suggest we use other-than-verbal methods from the beginning.

Sometimes, instead of seeing a client in the office we might take a walk along the beach, where we can enjoy the beauty of a sun-washed cove, smell the salt air, and be soothed by the rhythmic breaking of the waves upon the sand. Sometimes, without any need to discuss it, we both fall into a silent period of inner meditation. This is invariably a very nourishing experience for both of us, because *sharing* the experience is part of the nourishment. The informal atmosphere stimulates richer insights and generates more energy for their application.

At other times we might arrange to have lunch together after our session. Although this involves nourishment for the body, a far richer form of nourishment is taking place at the core of our inner selves. On other occasions we might experience the healing effects of laughter, or feel deeply moved by role-playing or dream therapy. We might also perform relaxation exercises or enjoy a fantasy together. In all these instances, the activities were merely avenues leading to a sense of greater closeness. Caring simply has to be experienced: love has to be shared and felt. When a relationship becomes more trusting and close, feelings of personal power increase and negative attitudes tend to lessen.

Also, I believe a professional helper comes to me, not as a sick man to a healer, or a beginning student to a teacher. I see our coming together as a joining of two equals, undertaking an adventure into areas of mystery. This means that we both begin in the dark, and we both must take some risks in order to find the path of the moment.

This sense of bonding together, of being willing to share the totality of my presence—my intellect, my senses, my body, my caring, my vulnerability as well as my strength—creates an environment in which the awful pain and occasional terror of loneliness are banished. It becomes an environment of actualization. Fears and negative attitudes which say "I can't" because they are dominated by the feeling, "I have to do it alone," are replaced with feelings of "I can" because they are complemented by feelings of "We can do it together."

Often the reality of this bonding can be questioned when fears generate within us. Yet the reality can frequently be restored by very small gestures. I have learned to trust my intuition in this regard. An inner sense will direct me to phone a client and share a few words of caring and concern. Or I might drop a brief note, or send a card or small gift, or share a recent book that I found interesting. Many times I have heard a professional client say, "I'm so happy you called. I was feeling very low and very much alone." In a few cases these contacts altered the movement of a person toward self-destruction. But in all cases it reminds both of us of the value and potency of our bonding. It gives us a new sense of closeness and warmth and a new perspective of our life-situation, as well as renewed hope for the future.

I remember my first visit to the Grand Canyon. I stood transfixed at the spot where I had my first full view of the canyon. When a friend suggested that I move just a few yards away I was reluctant, because I felt that such a small change of perspective would scarcely make a difference in my view.

How wrong I was! The new place gave me a radically different slant. I saw new rock formations and equally breathtaking colorations. I think it is very similar in therapy. We need a caring friend to be with us and at times suggest new ways of seeing old realities so that they become new realities for us.

A great deal of the art of self-caring centers around the experience of inner nourishment, and it is most often within a relationship that we come to our deepest sense of feeling nourished. This has an added quality of richness by reason of its mutuality, an aspect of great significance for professional clients. The awareness that in the very process of being nourished they are also nourishing develops a sense of worth and personal power. I find myself continually being nourished by these experiences, feeling new elation as a client and I come to new insights and feelings of strength, as we walk out of the maze into the light together. And I continue to discover ways of self-caring that I need to re-hear, re-learn and re-apply to my life.

A caring relationship supplies the nourishment for new growth. Professionals who begin to experience such a relationship note significant changes. They do not find it so hard to ask for help and to allow themselves to be cared for. Negative attitudes become easier to recognize and to alter. Fear tends to diminish, no longer thriving in darkness, but exposed to the light by a caring friend. And as the relationship deepens, new inner power creates feelings of confidence. Moments of laughter and touches of joy appear, slowly at first, but more consistently in time. Then new possibilities and alternatives emerge, like flowers in the desert after a spring rain, surprising us with their clarity and beauty. When this happens we have moved from powerlessness to power, from possibility to actualization.

We then begin to find ways of changing our present reality so that it becomes, in itself, a more productive and nourishing experience. At this point we have internalized the art of self-caring. We begin to listen to ourselves, our bodies and our inner needs, and we find ways to respond to what we hear. If it is something we can do for ourselves, by ourselves, we do it. If it is something that requires help from others, we admit it, and ask for that help. We have learned to care for ourselves, and to value the importance of this delicate art.

There is an ancient truth, "You cannot give what you do not have." For too long, professional caretakers have tried to care for others without adequately caring for themselves. The fact is we cannot care effectively for others when we are drained emotionally. We must learn the art of self-caring and view it as a life-long continuing education program.

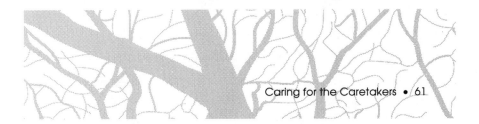

Then, as cared-for caretakers we can give to others the greatest gift of all: a caring person, refreshed, peaceful, ready to share the love of an abundant heart.

# CHAPTER EIGHT

## *We Can Go Home Again*

Nostalgia can be a terrible thing. During times of personal depression as well as during economic recession we have a powerful urge to remember "the good old days." We feel a desire to return to the innocence and dreams of childhood, when life was simpler and joys purer, and when adults took care of all our needs. Our desire to recapture the past as a way of overcoming the disappointment of the present often is an escape from responsibility. It represents a search for security and predictability by means of dependency on others. This siren call to childhood innocence is a myth, but it seems to be universal.

I remember a time when I was in Madrid. One warm Sunday in August I decided to visit some of the beautiful churches in the city. It happened to be a great feast day and First Communion ceremonies were taking place in a number of churches. In Spain these are elaborate affairs, resembling mini-weddings, in which the boys and girls, dressed in white, proceed in pairs accompanied by music and attendants. Later in the afternoon I saw elegant parties in my hotel with cakes and gifts for the children and wine and teas for their parents. A Spanish friend, commenting on this practice, said, "I think the real significance of these ceremonies is for the adults. It is a way for us to return to childhood and, for a moment, to recapture our lost innocence."

Such adventures in nostalgia may be touching for the moment, but they often leave us saddened and frustrated. Thomas Wolfe aptly reminds us of this in the title of his novel, *You Can't Go Home Again*. Going home, in this sense, is based on a false assumption. We assume that the past was perfect and unchanging. By going home we can recapture the goodness of the good old days and feel good again ourselves.

The reality is that the good old days were not all that good, and to try to recapture them is to deny the dynamism of life. Life is change, and this includes people and events and experiences and memories. Anyone who has ever returned to a home or school of childhood comes to realize this immediately. How small the desks in elementary schools are! Going home as a way of living out some dream or fantasy of the past, or of escaping from the pain of the present can never be a satisfying experience. We can't go home in this sense.

There is, however, a way in which we can return to the past in order to bring the richness of the past into the present and help us move more securely into the future. By getting in touch with our past history so that we feel empowered by it, we are able to transfer the beauty and vitality of past experience into our present and future life

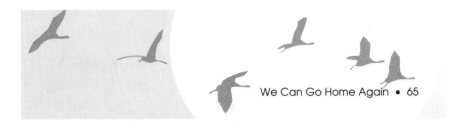

situations. We discover new ways of seeing and sensing ourselves, and we behold new options for our lives.

Alex Haley shows us the wonderful effects of this kind of going home experience. His book, *Roots*, not only recounts the wealth of information that he acquired about his past history, but also reveals the dramatic impact that his search had on his future life. It has inspired many others to seek out their own personal roots.

Understanding our personal connection with past culture and tradition can be very important for us, especially when available early in life. Today in Hawaii children are fortunate to be growing up at a time of great renaissance of Hawaiian history and culture. Hawaiian music, language, chant and dance are introduced at the elementary school level, and students become proficient by high school. It is inspiring to see large numbers of young men and women spending long hours after school learning the art and discipline of the ancient hula, for which there are annual high school competitions. *Kupunas,* or elders, visit schools regularly to "talk story" and share the collected memories of the early Hawaiians. The beauty and power of the past traditions provide a combination of the practical and ideal, of material skills and spiritual beliefs. This marvelous blend empowers young people to create a balance between past and present in their own lives.

Going home in this sense, as a future-related experience, can be an extremely satisfying, even transcendent, life-changing experience. But it demands a certain kind of humility. We must return to the past with no preconceived notions of what we will find. We have to have the eyes and attitudes of a child. This means letting go of our dreams, of surrendering our expectations. Frances Horn in her book, *I Want One Thing*, says:

> *I concentrate entirely on getting to this place of **willingness**. It means letting go of the hold on the specific outcome I had wanted, and allowing myself to open to WHATEVER outcome might be appropriate in the circumstances.*

This letting go of our dreams permits what Eastern philosophers call "beginner's mind"—the one condition essential for true learning. With this type of openness we may discover not only something different from our dream, but often something far better.

I experienced this when, as an adult, I returned to the campus of Notre Dame University. As a child I had first visited it with my parents. That first visit was in early summer, and the campus was filled with lush greenness: lawns, shrubs, and heavy-leafed trees. I was enchanted by the beauty of the place and the hospitality of the priests and brothers. Attending Notre Dame some day became a dream. However, a world war and the need to earn a living made this an impossible dream for me.

Years later I was invited to conduct a workshop for some of the faculty at Notre Dame, and I found myself thinking of the campus with nostalgia, hoping perhaps to recapture some of that past enchantment. But this time my arrival was in mid-summer. The grass was brown, the weather humid, the leaves were thin and turning yellow, and the campus seemed much smaller. I realized that I had to let go of the dream which I had been nourishing since childhood if I were to make my present experience a new discovery.

The gift that I received in exchange was a discovery that has continued to enrich my life. I found that my original dream had associated Notre Dame with a place where *I would be taught*. My second visit revealed the value of *learning that is shared*. Since I felt very much at home at Notre Dame, I was especially open and responsive to the faculty, and they in turn helped to create an

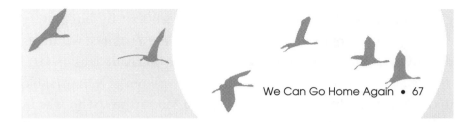

environment in which we all taught and learned from one another. This concept has become a valued treasure for me in the ensuing years. My original dream pales in comparison to the later discovery.

Dreams tend to color the past too vividly. They resemble the first color television sets, which gave people faces that were either too orange or too green. We tend to paint the past in similar distortions of brightness. Dreams also seem to stop time and freeze memories at past moments. We then become prisoners of our own fixed images, rather than free spirits enjoying the changing colors reflected from the sun-splashed prism. We need something of this fluid attitude as we return to past events and situations, if we are to see new aspects and colorations.

One of the reasons we find it difficult to let go of our dreams is our need for predictability. When the present is disappointing and the future appears bleak or frightening because it is unknown, we may seek security in the past, where things seem more predictable. However, predictability is a two-edged sword. It can be a source of reassurance, but it can also be a rut in which we become stuck. Within us we have a counter-need for adventure and spontaneity. We are delighted by loving and joyful surprises. The challenge for us is to take the risk of *letting go of our dreams without feeling overwhelmed by our fear of the unknown.*

Sometimes it helps if we can find some aspect of the experience that is predictable. This can function as a base of security for us. It is then easier to permit ourselves to be open to new discoveries. This process also teaches us the importance of not getting caught in extremes or polarities. We come to realize that not all of the past is good nor all the future frightening. We learn that by integrating different aspects of an experience we can create a balance within us that gives us the self-confidence to face difficult challenges.

Helen Hayes, the actress, is an example of a woman who was able to do this in her life. She married Charlie MacArthur, who was in many ways very different from her. Helen was shy and serious and Charlie was a charming, lovable clown. He was anything but predictable. Before their marriage he said, "Helen, I may never be able to give you contentment, but you'll never be bored."

Their relationship was marked by moments of ecstasy and times of tragedy. Charlie's depressions and drinking bouts, as well as the death of their daughter, Mary, cast long shadows across their life together. Yet, amidst the darkness and the turbulence, Helen was able, with Charlie's help, to hold on to the one aspect of his personality that was predictable: his unswerving love and devotion to her. It became Helen's Rock of Gibraltar, something to cling to and be supported by. And Charlie consistently found ways to put Helen back in touch with that vital life-force between them. When they were physically separated, their memories formed a way for them to return to the past, to go home again, and to call forth the power of a living, present relationship. An example of this is a letter that Charlie wrote to Helen from London in 1943, after many years of married life together:

> *Angel:*
> *It's 5:30 AM and I've given up the idea of sleep so I might as well be writing you a letter. I've been alternately reading bad plays and thinking pleasantly of you and wishing you were here in my arms. I've been remembering so many things, from our buggy ride to Fraunces Tavern on down the years—all my boobish love antics return to entertain me. I run upstairs in East 40th Street with you in my arms... I see you coming down Madison avenue in a little gray suit with a green orchid I sent you, on your shoulder...And the first time I kissed you in a cab and how you lied ever after when you said*

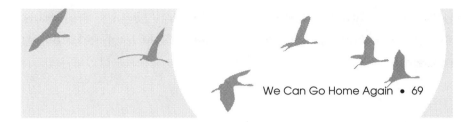

*you didn't lean toward me first. And sitting with you in Childs and going over the brow of yon hills in France…And the time you got tight and were so gay at Barney Glazer's…And now I'll go to work. Don't worry about me. I hope I always have this particular form of insomnia. Thank you for a very pleasant night, my dearest, only love. All this is so little of my happiness.*
*Charlie*

It was this form of "going home" that enabled Helen to balance her need for stability with the fact of Charlie's unpredictable ways. These memories put Helen in touch with the depth and vibrancy of the love that united them, supplying the strength to meet the growing demands on her personal and professional life.

This is bringing the power of the past into the present and making it available to us for the future. But "going home" in the sense of escaping from current problems by dwelling on past joys or successes, makes us prisoners of the past. It leaves us feeling frustrated and unsatisfied, if not discouraged. This type of going home experience is a flight from reality that seeks shelter in the pseudo-safety and dependency of childhood.

If we choose to release our fixed dream of the past, returning instead to seek insights and power for our future, we discover a genuine treasure in the experience. Through contact with our roots, whether it be our immediate past or past culture and tradition, we can be given the gift of seeing ourselves in a new way. Like the prism turning in the sun, we may see new colors and aspects of inner beauty that were hidden to us. We may see untapped talents. We may feel a new surge of inner power and self-esteem, released from deep reservoirs within us. And we will most likely begin to sense new ways of connecting the vitality of the past with the hope and promise of the future.

# CHAPTER NINE

## *The Loss that Is Gain*

One of my earliest childhood memories centers around being lost. The experience took place in a supermarket when I was about three years old. Fascinated by the array of colorful things on the shelves, I wandered away from my mother. After a period of exploration I suddenly became aware that I was surrounded by unfamiliar faces and my mother was nowhere in sight. With mounting panic I ran up and down the aisles searching for her, but in vain. I remember stopping and thinking, "She has gone home. She has forgotten me."

With that thought came the sinking feeling of loss—a mixture of terror and despair. All I could do was sit and sob until finally my mother discovered me, dried my tears and reassured me that I had not been abandoned. Although that incident took place many years ago, I can still recall very clearly the pain of that experience of loss.

It would be many years before I would learn the mystery of loss, its relationship with gain, and its value as a teacher. Now I can appreciate the fact that life often presents us an invitation to awareness by means of painful experiences such as loss. I have come to see that, in life, things are seldom black and white, all good or all bad, but rather a blending of both aspects. Asian philosophers teach us that only when we can accept and integrate both the positive and negative aspects of an experience can we attain the balance that results in inner peace. I believe they are right.

I also believe we have inner wisdom. This "higher" part of ourselves knows what is important for our growth. At times it draws us toward painful experiences so that certain needed changes can be made. I have noticed this happening in my own life and in the lives of my clients. It strikes me as more than coincidence that so many people will confess that some of their best life-learnings and transformations have occurred as a result of painful experiences, some often involving a sense of loss.

In examining these experiences, it seems that feelings of loss trigger feelings of hopelessness, helplessness and powerlessness. These are the initial feelings. As the experience of loss is understood in its totality we find that for each aspect of loss there is a counterbalancing aspect of gain. The challenge for us is to be aware of this *at the onset* of a loss experience.

The first step in making loss a productive growth experience is the recognition that the initial pain need not spell ultimate disaster. The second step is to gradually let go of any fixed ideas we may have about the experience and its significance in our life. These two steps permit us to be open to new awareness and new learning. From these come the actual gain for our lives.

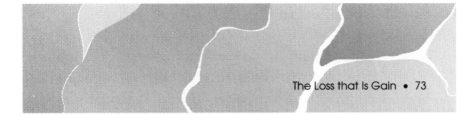

I discovered the importance of these steps some years ago when my home was burglarized. Among other things, I lost a fine stereo set. I did not replace the stereo immediately, and in the interim I became aware of the value of good music in my life. Before that, I had simply taken it for granted; since then I have been more consciously grateful for its gift. This was part of the gain from my loss. There was another, more significant one.

At some point after the theft I became aware that I had also permitted the thieves to steal my inner peace. I was holding on to anger and resentment over the violation of my home and the theft of my possessions. Clinging to these negative feelings reinforced my sense of loss. When, finally, I became aware of what I was doing, I chose to reclaim my inner peace. Through meditation and prayer I let go of the things that were stolen and forgave the persons involved. I reminded myself that these articles were really only on loan to me from a loving universe and I could pass them on. They would be replaced by others in due time. With this gesture of release I was suddenly free from the resentment. I regained my inner peace. It was a valuable lesson for me. The loss as well as the gain were both important parts of a growth experience.

A friend of mine described similar learnings from the loss of a job in his youth. He told me that being fired, although a terrible blow to his ego, was the best thing that ever happened to him. He might have remained an accountant for the rest of his life. Getting fired gave him an opportunity to return to college and ultimately find a new career as a counselor, for which he is gifted by nature. He is an effective counselor and finds it a very rewarding career. His loss, painful and embarrassing, was also an invitation to new awareness and the source of new gain.

Loss and gain are also bound together in one of life's most painful experiences—the death of a loved one. What is at first so devastating can become the invitation to new values and direction. We often begin to re-examine our lives, and rearrange our priorities.

This happened in my own life. The sudden death of my sister in an automobile accident left me stunned. After the grief, I began to reflect on the brevity of her life and on plans she had made that could not be completed. Then I saw a parallel in my own life. With this awareness I began to focus my energy on living more in the present moment than in the past or the future. I started noticing things: clouds, birds, sunsets, the smell of the sea breeze, the warmth in a glance, the love in a touch. Then a marvelous thing happened: I lost my fear of death. It was as if the more I began to live life, the less reason I had to worry about the last stage of life. My initial loss was extremely painful, but the ensuing gain was a whole new sense of the meaning of life itself.

Loss of "the dream" is a painful life experience for many people in mid-life. The dream represents some fixed idea or belief upon which we hang our hopes for happiness. In mid-life we begin to realize that the dream is not going to find expression in our lives. We come to see that we will not be president of the company, or find the perfect lover, or be a famous artist. Then the sense of loss can become very real and very painful. Yet gain interweaves here too.

A friend of mine faced this challenge when he was nearing forty. He hated his job, his marriage was a bitter yoke, and his future was gloomy. His dream of being successful in that particular career and in that particular relationship had proved unrealistic.

Once he recognized and accepted this fact, he could begin to let go of the dream. New energy became available as he released himself from his self-imposed burden. He began to see alternatives, and these generated new enthusiasm to replace his pessimistic outlook.

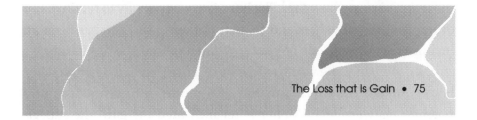

He and his wife agreed that a divorce was really best for both of them. He quit his job and moved to another city.

Today he is doing work that he enjoys, and he is involved in a relationship that is supportive and energizing. His apparent loss of the dream moved him to let go of an illusion, and his gain was a new life that was even better than the dream.

This experience demonstrates how tenaciously we can cling to myths which are actually self-destructive. We grasp a belief or hold on to a pattern of behavior as if our very salvation depended on it. Robert Frost, in his poem *Mending Wall,* reminds us of this tendency as he describes neighboring farmers who, each spring, go out to mend the stone wall that separates them. Frost wonders why they need this wall. He finds his answer in the unquestioning acceptance by the farmer of his father's saying, "Good fences make good neighbors."

I think this is true for many of us. From childhood on through adult life we pick up bits and pieces of beliefs and behaviors which become a part of our personal folklore. We then cling to them and defend them vigorously, like a drowning person fighting off a rescuer. True, it takes great courage to let go of our treasured myths and risk an unknown possibility. But it is equally true that it actually takes less energy to let go of something than to hold on to it. And often it is the gesture of opening one's hand, of reaching out to another person, that externalizes the opening of one's heart to a new way of life.

One of the most beautiful examples of a person who has learned the lesson of loss and gain is a friend of mine in Japan. This woman, in her seventies, has seen many of her old beliefs altered throughout the war and post-war years. She has discovered a way to retain many of her traditional values and to adapt others. And she has been an inspiration to hundreds of young women whom she has taught.

Not long ago, she wrote to tell me of a fire that had destroyed her home outside Tokyo. In a matter of minutes, fifty years of family possessions were lost. Yet her letter indicated the gain she experienced. She wrote, "After my initial grief over the loss of many dear things, I was surprised to discover, as well, a feeling of relief. I think I had become a prisoner of my possessions instead of their owner. Losing them somehow freed me. I had enjoyed them and loved having them—and now no longer need them. I am free to gather new things and to seek new paths in my life."

This remarkable woman has since found a new career after retirement from a teaching position at a university. She is currently involved in training women to be para-professional counselors, a rather innovative activity for Japanese women. In letting go of her possessions, she was freed to put new energy into a new career. Her loving generosity touches the lives of many people, and as one who has been touched by her caring, I can only be grateful for the loss that has proved to be such a gain for her.

I find at this point in my life that I tend to view loss more as an opportunity than a misfortune. I do not enjoy the pain, but I understand it better. I now begin to look for the message behind the pain sooner than I did before. I also am aware that the experience of loss often has a refining effect on my personality. It can soften the rough edges of my judgments and smooth the troubled waters of my angry feelings. It can, in addition, sharpen my sense of compassion for others who are in pain and confusion. So while I do not welcome the painful aspect of loss, I am better able to appreciate it as *a necessary part of my growth*. This awareness makes it easier to try to open myself to new learning and needed changes. Sometimes I even succeed!

This paradox of interwoven loss and gain is not new. Philosophers and saints have long referred to it as one of the central

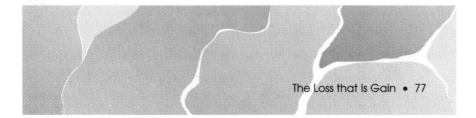

mysteries of life. Long ago Saint Paul wrote, "I count everything as loss compared to the gain of knowing Christ." What is needed, however, is to translate the concept into practical application for our personal lives.

Living is the essence of life. Whenever we hold on to the pain of loss we stop living, and our energy moves into self-destructive forms of existence. We settle for barely surviving and cling to unrealistic attitudes and expectations. Letting go of loss enables us to start living again. It releases energy for rebirth and new life. But *first* we must let go of loss in order to receive the gain of getting on with life.

And ultimately, that is what really matters; getting on with life. Sometimes when we are in great pain we are tempted to give up the struggle, or to withdraw into the shadows and lick our wounds. The only thing that will give us renewed strength is the realization that we must put our loss behind us, accept the lessons to be learned, open ourselves to the gain, and get on with life. Robert Frost sums it up for us in another of his poems, Stopping By Woods on a Snowy Evening:

The woods are lovely, dark and deep
But I have promises to keep
And miles to go before I sleep
And miles to go before I sleep.

# CHAPTER TEN

## *Fixing or Fostering*

There is in most of us a deep need to fix things, to make them right. We like to see things well-ordered, properly working. And nowhere is this need more apparent then in men and women who enter the helping professions.

I am one of those persons. Like many in my profession, I have sought to promote the health and growth of my clients; and I believe I have done this with a fair degree of success and satisfaction. I have always been aware of my desire to help people, but only recently have I become aware that I also harbor a hidden need to "fix" them.

The awareness of this hidden need came as a shock to me,

for I had prided myself on being a person-centered counselor, more concerned with facilitating growth than directing it. My first awakening came one day when I reflected upon my frustration with a particular client. Handsome, well-dressed, successful, this man felt trapped in a very destructive marriage, yet he seemed to be unwilling to seek a divorce. Suddenly a gentle inner voice spoke to me. "He is not ready to leave his wife. It is your desire rather than his. You think you know what is best for him." I then realized that despite my pretense of wanting to help this man, I was more intent on trying to "fix" him.

This experience was very sobering for me. It taught me, first of all, how blind we can be to these hidden needs. It also led me to trace the roots of this desire to fix things to my early childhood training. Finally, I was able to recognize the hidden face of arrogance in my assumption that I know what is best for others.

My early training centered on "doing things correctly." I learned that clothes had to be placed on hangers or folded neatly and placed in a drawer. Broken things had to be mended, mistakes needed to be corrected. There was a right way and a wrong way to do all of these things, and I was rewarded when I chose the right way.

In the positive sense I was learning responsibility, but this lesson was heavily contaminated by perfectionism. My mother had been reared in a tradition which boasted, "Her kitchen is so clean you could eat off the linoleum floor." In later life she suffered a stroke and her physician needed to lecture her, "Right now there are some things you cannot do. For instance, you have to let dust accumulate on these tables and say, 'to hell with it.'" My mother pondered this for a moment and quietly replied, "I don't know if I can do that." Her obsession with having a "perfect" home and doing things the "right way" got transferred to me very early.

There were many telltale signs sprinkled across the path of my childhood and young adulthood, but at the time I saw these as indications of self-discipline rather than perfectionism. I was proud

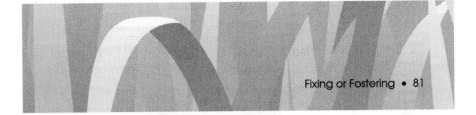

of the fact that I kept my room tidy, made my bed as soon as I got up, put things away when I was finished with them. No cluttered desks or messy cabinets for me: I had files for notes, indexes for books, and records of all important matters.

I am sure that others were aware of my incipient perfectionism. When I was in graduate school I lived in a one-bedroom apartment with a very decent fellow—who was also rather untidy. We came to a gentlemen's agreement about keeping things in some semblance of order. He agreed to keep the living room area neat since that was what visitors saw, and I agreed to let him maintain disorder in his part of the bedroom.

The arrangement worked very well until one afternoon, when he and a mutual friend of ours returned from the beach and tracked sand from the front door to the bedroom. My roommate received a rather harsh scolding from me, and some time later told me that when the visitor left he referred to us as "the odd couple." In the TV situation comedy of the same name, one of the roommates is sloppy and the other obsessively tidy. This comparison left me feeling insulted and misunderstood.

Another aspect of my early training which propelled me along the perfectionistic path was my devotion to the Catholic tradition. I was taught that I am my brother's keeper, that I have a responsibility to care for others in need, and that the greatest law is that of charity. This neatly dovetailed into my belief that things have to be fixed. Now it became people who needed to be fixed. I was preparing myself for entry into one of the helping professions, although these might be better described as the "fixing" professions.

For a number of years I was very successful. Clients who needed a loving father or a gentle guide flocked to me and let me fix them to our mutual satisfaction. Yet even then there was an undercurrent of unease inside me. Not all clients welcomed my paternal ministrations or valued my indirect direction. They sensed the iron hand hidden in the velvet glove, and many resisted or resented it. And curiously enough, at this time I was advocating the "person-centered" approach, which values the inner wisdom of the client rather than the therapist. What I supported in theory I abrogated in practice.

As occasionally happens to people in the helping professions, one of my clients became my teacher, and helped open my eyes to the reality of my behavior. One day this particular client said to me quite directly, "You are disappointed with me, aren't you?" There was no way I could evade the truth and so I answered, "Yes, I am." The young man then said to me, "You know, you have been pushing me too hard and I simply cannot move at the pace of your expectations for me. I have to find my own pace, and *you* have to walk at *my* pace or you cannot help me."

This eloquent summary of our relationship made it possible for me to begin to see the pattern of my expectations and assumptions. Gradually I was able to let go of my need to fix this client. I accepted his invitation, and found that walking at his pace was as rewarding for me as it was therapeutic for him. And when it was time for us to end the counseling relationship, I told him how much he had given me by that one remark. It seemed to him a fair exchange, and to this day we have remained good friends.

My greatest surprise was to discover the subtlety of this need to fix things and people. While I genuinely believed I was being altruistic, loving, and other-centered, I was actually being self-centered and self-serving. Despite the fact that I knew people do not like to be told what to do or where to go, I found myself gently but perseveringly edging them in the direction I felt was best for them. Although they were telling me in many nonverbal ways that they wanted to fix themselves, I somehow managed to discount these messages.

I suspect there will always be a trace of "father knows best" in me, especially with clients who have had a tradition of being dependent on parents, teachers, coaches and counselors. But at least I am more sensitive to this possibility, and hear inner bells ringing whenever I sense feelings of disappointment.

Today I am more comfortable with the fact that people have their own rhythms and their own individual schedules in life. I am somewhat less arrogant concerning notions of what is best for another person. Experience tells me over and over that even things we term "disasters" at one point are later seen as blessings. Many of us can learn valuable life-lessons only "the hard way"—through mistaken judgments, suffering and apparent failure. As a result I am more at ease with clients who are slow to learn and slower to change.

I am reminded of the story of Barry Neil Kaufman, author of *Son Rise*, who helped his son to emerge from years of autism. One day he realized that he and his wife, indirectly, had been saying to his son, "You are not O.K. You must change." Kaufman decided that he was going to give his son a different message, one which would say, "You are O.K. and I love you as you are. You are doing the best you can." I was tremendously impressed by this idea. This message is precisely what we all want to hear from others—no scolding, or correction, or being lectured about "right" ways to act, but rather understanding, compassion and encouragement. Today I find it easier to believe that clients are "doing the best they can." With help and encouragement they may be able to change and improve, but that is *their* choice and it must be done according to *their own* inner impulses.

I prefer the concept of *change* to fixing. Fixing implies something is broken to begin with; it carries the connotation of wrong and leads to guilt. When we feel we have done something that is wrong we waste valuable energy by engaging in interior monologues of self-scolding. However, we *change* something we do not like without this inner punishment. When the sun is too bright for our eyes, we change to dark glasses. When we discover we are overweight we change our diet and exercise routine. And when we are exhausted physically and emotionally we can change our inner feelings by sharing a sunset and a lovely meal with a caring friend. Change focuses on newness, on re-birth and renewal. It is an essential part of the life process and it is entirely natural to us. By emphasizing a need for and a desire to change rather than fixing something that is wrong, we allow our creative energy to build and facilitate the actual change.

With every movement toward change there is a counter move-ment triggered by fear. The risk of the unknown activates our fantasies and expands our anxiety. And it is in precisely this area that I, as a counselor, can do my best work. Clients do not need my advice, nor my correction. They do need my support and encouragement so that they can regain their slipping self-confidence and restore their former courage. People need reassurance that they are doing the best they can, and that I support them in any change they choose to make. With this kind of assistance they can release the imprisoning chains of fear and liberate their creative resources. *Fostering* such as this enables individuals to arrange for their own "fixing."

Occasionally a person will be so frightened of accepting respon-sibility that dependency appears preferable, and manipulation be-comes inevitable. A counselor needs to listen very carefully, to pick up both messages the client sends: "I need you" and "Please don't let me get away with this." Ultimately, such a person is hoping to outgrow the fearful child and become a mature adult, and the counselor sometimes has to offer "tough love" by avoiding the manipulations of the client.

I recall a young woman who came to this point in our counseling relationship. Very attractive, she would wear a new dress and ask if

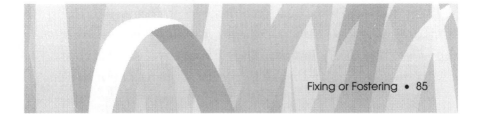

I thought it pretty. She changed her hairstyle, perfume, and make-up. She would tell me how much she favored the shirts I wore. All of these were attention-getting gestures. There was even a touching quality apart from a hint of seductiveness. She was like a little girl seeking her father's approval.

I confronted her with my observations of her behavior, adding, "I appreciate the beauty of the woman you want to be too much to encourage you to continue to act as a needy little girl. I want to help you to become that strong, beautiful woman." She reacted with anger saying, "Well, it's clear to me you don't understand me at all. I think I'll have to find another counselor." I responded, "Perhaps you are right. I may have done as much as I can for you. If you wish I can recommend a couple of other counselors."

The woman did not follow through with her threat. She admitted her behavior had been both seductive and childish, since it was part of an old pattern for her. A few months later when our sessions were finished, she sent me a card of appreciation. The card was a crazy contemporary design. The outside showed a picture of a little baby, mouth open, screaming: "I want you! I need you! I have to have you, you, YOU!" On the inside was the same child, composed, sucking his finger, and saying, "If I can't have you, can I have a fire engine...or a cookie?" Apparently both of us had got the message.

We cannot fix another person. When we try to do so that person resists and resents our efforts. The only person I can fix is myself, and that is no small task, but rather a lifetime challenge. However, I can support and foster the growth of others; I can be with them as they face new challenges for change, joining with them in overcoming their fears.

Nor do I have to be perfect in order to perform well. This truth applies to everyone: *Even when we are weak and frightened we can help each other*. Together, joining hands and hearts, we can find courage to overcome our fears and make important changes in our lives.

# CHAPTER ELEVEN

# *A Time for Doing*

One day, as I was listening to a client describe her problems in some detail, I became aware that her story telling was really a disguised cry for help. She felt trapped in her life situation, helpless to alter it, but also afraid to confront it openly. That session taught me a valuable lesson. I discovered that telling a story is often the way people approach solutions to personal problems. But for many persons, story telling becomes a hindrance to the kind of awareness that precedes change and growth.

This is a common occurrence in many counseling relationships. After a number of sessions and some impressive growth, a client reaches a plateau. We continue to meet and the client continues his or her story telling, but there is little if any movement. Like a mountain climber, the person works hard on the initial ascent, and welcomes a place to rest for awhile. Then, surveying the difficulty of scaling the remaining peak the climber becomes anxious. A glance down at the sheer drop below may even induce terror. Story telling becomes a way in which the client can stay in the safe place with a trusted companion. At the same time, however one can feel just as trapped on the plateau as at the beginning of the sessions. Story telling also can be a hidden plea for help, saying in effect: "Please take my hand and support me as I continue the ascent!"

Now aware of this hidden cry, I am better able to respond by gently interrupting the narrative and re-directing the focus. I might ask the client to be aware of what is happening in his or her body at that moment. We might do a few breathing exercises to reduce tension. Often the client will experience a new flow of energy through the body. Sometimes the interruption takes the form of an invitation to dramatize a part of the story by means of role-playing together.

The change in tone from story telling is frequently remarkable. Instead of mere recital of events, eyes flash with anger. The voice quivers with remembered pain. If I over-dramatize some part, the client might break into laughter at my interpretation. These interruptions permit us to join hands, to move from the plateau, and to continue the ascent of the mountain. After we make progress together I often share a story that illustrates what happens on the plateau.

As a young man I spent some time in Mexico. One day friends invited me to join them in driving out to the pyramids, a little distance from Mexico City. After exploring these ancient monuments, Maria, the very attractive daughter of this family, said to me, "Let's climb to the top. There is a wonderful view from the sacrificial altar there." I agreed and we made our climb up very steep and narrow

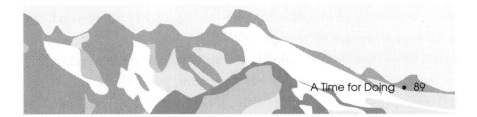

stone steps. When I reached the top and stood on the small sacrificial stone I looked out over a vast panorama. It was beautiful.

Then I made the mistake of looking down at the spot where the family was waiting, and I froze. In the excitement of the adventure I had forgotten about my acrophobia. For several moments I experienced sheer terror, fantasizing about remaining on top of that pyramid for the remainder of my life. My catastrophic expectations were interrupted by Maria's voice, saying, "I think we should go back down now."

The interruption moved me from my focus on powerlessness. I realized I had to *do* something. In a flash of inspiration born of desperate need I said to Maria, as convincingly as possible, "Look, Maria, the descent is very treacherous because of the narrow footings. I suggest we go down very slowly, and I am going to hold on to your hand very tightly to make sure you don't slip." Shameful as my dishonesty was, it was the only way my masculine pride would permit me to ask for help. Joining hands with Maria I felt enough combined strength to move from my plateau.

Something similar occurs in counseling when clients use story telling to remain on the plateau. I remember one man whom I confronted with this pattern. Even after an interruption he would return immediately to another narrative. My confrontation came as a surprise, upsetting him to the point of tears. Finally he was able to tell me that his initial growth had been wonderful and he was very grateful for my help. But when he began to fall back into old patterns of behavior, he feared that I would be disappointed and reject him as his parents had once done. Story telling was his way to be with me while avoiding greater risks. Yet he was genuinely relieved when I confronted him with this pattern.

Talking with a counselor is a way in which people frequently come to new experiences of inner worth and personal power. As the relationship deepens, trust is built, fear is discarded and growth is enhanced. But talking *with* is quite different from talking *about*. Talking about, or story telling, permits the speaker to act as a spectator to the events discussed rather than an involved participant. Responsibility can be avoided, and since the emphasis is on relating a tale which is not new, there is little openness to transformative insights and awareness. With story telling the client becomes more of a teacher than a student. Unfortunately this approach leads to frustration and greater confusion.

My own experience with this phenomenon was validated when I attended a Gestalt workshop with the late Fritz Perls. I was amazed at how effective his frequent interruptions of story telling were. At first I could not see a connection between his drawing the client's attention to a twitching foot and the problem they both were examining. But soon I realized that the twitching foot was telling the real story. Fritz often said, "The body doesn't lie," and I saw this confirmed each day during the workshop. The client's words might be measured and the tone of voice controlled, but the body was telling a story of discomfort, anxiety and deep fear. Having the client focus on the bodily movements would often cause those hidden feelings to surface so that they could be expressed openly. The words alone conveyed distortion, but the words along with the language of the body communicated the truth. Saint-Exupery's line from *The Little Prince* has much wisdom: "Words are the source of misunderstandings."

Fritz Perls helped me to see that the client is often caught in a bind. He or she wants to unload the burden of guilt and inner pain but is also afraid to do so. He or she wants help, but is not brave enough to ask for it. The person wants to surrender control, to stop his or her verbal ramblings, but fears that he or she will fly out of

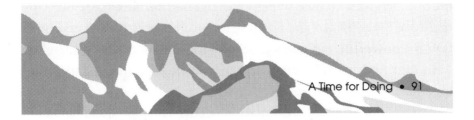

control completely. The counselor, hearing this double message, can gently lead the client from talking about to doing.

Over the years I have become more creative with various forms of narrative interruption. I began using this approach with counselors who came to me for help with their own problems. Realizing that we both were very articulate, I asked for permission to utilize other forms of interaction, and they readily agreed. As a result our sessions were very spontaneous. After some talking together, I might suggest spending some quiet time together by the sea, listening to the surf and watching the hungry seagulls. Or we might do some calisthenics or share a fantasy together. The addition of the non-verbal interactions tended to shift the person's focus from a negative experience of the problem to their growing feelings of resourcefulness.

Later I had occasion to spend weekends with clients and found the approach working productively in this setting also. One friend's marriage was in jeopardy. He wanted to do some counseling while enjoying the healing effects of sun and sea. I picked him up at the airport on a Friday evening and for several hours he talked about his anguished experience at home.

Before turning in we spent a few moments by the sea, soothed by the gentle winds and the beauty of the starry night. We slept well that night, and the following day I invited my friend to do things instead of talking about the marriage. I felt it was important to relax, to play and be nourished before attacking the marriage problems. By late afternoon, my friend was relaxed and laughing, and in this setting we began our formal counseling session. At one point, I interrupted his narrative to suggest re-enacting a recent dream. This method opened the door to an awareness which changed his life. He experienced the reality of his behavior and attitude toward his wife for the first time. It was a powerful, moving experience for him, and later counseling with him and his wife enabled them to build a new relationship together.

This remarkable transformation occurred in the short period of a day and a half, during a very brief counseling session. As I pondered over this I realized that although there was little formal counseling, there was a constant sharing. We did many things together, formal and informal, significant and pedestrian. We experienced each other in many new ways, deepening the sort of intimacy which fosters trust and a willingness to take new risks.

I also experimented with this approach on weekends designed for couples. Besides learning communication skills and discussing their problems, they did a great many things together, from tasks to play. They learned to bake bread and prepare gourmet meals. They gathered strawberries from the garden and turned them into delicious ice cream. Roles disappeared, and the kitchen was filled with laughter as well as the smell of bread baking. When the time came for formal discussions, the atmosphere was very different from previous group sessions with couples. These men and women were more open and willing to learn about themselves and to accept responsibility for changes that needed to be made in their lives. *Sharing-by-doing* helped to make the *sharing-by-talking* a deeper and more productive experience for everyone.

Since those weekends I have used the approach of doing things together in a variety of ways. I have done art work with clients. We have painted fences and repaired leaky faucets. We have prepared and shared picnic lunches. We have done ceramic work and made mango chutney. We have done exercises, body movement and dance, foot massage and Shiatsu. We have planted bulbs in the fall and shared the blooms in the spring. Often during our work sessions a client would pause and share a very profound insight that may

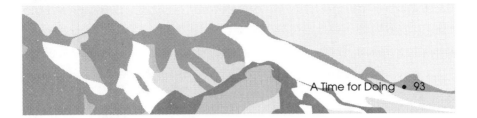

have touched him or her deeply. As a result of these many different shared experiences, the counseling relationship became more of a mutual experience than merely talking ever was. At some tasks the client had greater skill than I and became the teacher. I became more relaxed, spontaneous and creative, and people experienced me more fully, freely and lovingly as a consequence.

I do not want to suggest that we never discussed important life issues. We did. But we dealt with these issues *after* we had done things together, and *while* doing things together. The priority was and is on sharing a new creative experience, of developing a sense of camaraderie from working and playing together.

It is also important to note that this approach may not be suited to every client, or may not be appropriate for a client at a particular time. Some people prefer talking, and with these I share talking and listening. Intuition seems to be the best guide in making this determination.

Most of us, like clams, jealously guard our inner sanctums, and protect ourselves from outside forces that would try to pry us open. We will not be forced to share ourselves with outsiders. However, like clams placed in the sun, when we experience the continued warmth of a caring relationship, we relax and from within open ourselves to added warmth and greater growth. Doing things together can provide this sunny warm environment for us.

# CHAPTER TWELVE

# *The Inner Wise Man*

Carl Jung said that each person has a "wise man" in the depths of his or her soul. The concept does not refer to a male figure, but is a metaphor for the source of wisdom and healing which resides in each one of us. Today we are discovering a variety of ways to gain access to that precious inner source. Intuition is one of those ways.

I have come to appreciate and value the importance of intuition in all areas of my life, but especially in my work as a counselor. When I was young and just beginning the work of counseling, I was very anxious to help people. But I was ignorant of the art of counseling. I felt that I had many answers for clients and I was eager for them to come to me so that I might give them advice and help them solve their problems. However, I discovered that this approach did not work very well. Many would listen to me, thank me for the advice, leave and never return!

Then I met Carl Rogers and began a long association with him which changed my life and my counseling. I learned so much from him simply by being in his presence and observing him interact with other people. I learned more from him in that way than I did from books or other teachers. I would watch Carl Rogers working with people, listening to them, being so very patient with them, and I would think to myself, "Why doesn't he tell them what to do?" But Dr. Rogers would offer no advice, no direction. Instead he looked at them with great loving compassion and listened to them with an open heart. This somehow touched their hearts also.

I realized that the Rogers approach was a very effective way of interacting with another person. He was doing more than listening to the problem about the marriage or the children or the boss. He was listening to something underneath that external problem. Listening with the heart, he was hearing feelings which represented the impact of that problem upon the person. If, for instance, the client was a parent talking about problems with a child, Dr. Rogers might be hearing the emotion of fear, and he would respond by saying, "I sense that you are very frightened about what might happen to your child." The heart of the parent would usually be touched, making it easier to talk openly about the inner fears.

I came to see that the real problems were not the external situations being discussed. The real problems were the inner fears, self-doubts and hidden guilts. Carl Rogers heard these problems of the heart because he was listening with his heart.

I also discovered that this listening is not easy. My own ego and my desire to appear important in the eyes of others often prevented me from listening with the heart. It was not until I learned to be more humble as a person and a counselor that I could listen more with my

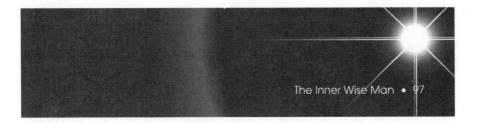

heart than my head. Then I found I could turn off the part of my mind that said, "This is the answer to the problem." I could *change my focus from the problem to the person,* and hear a different message. I could hear something besides the words—the inner anguish and inner fears which were paralyzing the client. This was the beginning of my being able to listen with the heart. It was also the awakening and releasing of my intuition.

My counseling changed radically. When a client would come to me and talk about various problems I would listen to those things, but I became more sensitive to the sound of the voice, to the rapid or hesitant speech, to the movement or rigidity of the body. And sometimes, as I was listening with the heart, an image would appear in my mind. If I reported this image to the client I would often discover that the image had a very significant meaning to the client.

For example, a counselor once came seeking help with his personal problems. Once again I discovered that psychologists have the same problems as everyone else: marriage problems, family problems, sexual problems, even communication problems. This particular counselor came to discuss an unhappy marriage relationship. But as I listened with my heart, I heard a great undertone of sadness. Next, an unusual image appeared in my mind. I pictured a small boy on a red bicycle, riding very fast, his hair flying in the wind and a smile of happiness on his face.

Now, one thing I have learned about intuition is that you never censor the information which comes to you, whether it is a feeling or an image. You don't make a judgment: "That is silly"; "That image doesn't make sense." You avoid any judgment. The reason is that intuition is not subject to rational analysis. It comes from another part of our mind and speaks to us in symbols at times, as our dreams often speak to us. So, I did not try to understand or interpret the boy on the red bicycle. I simply reported it to the client, saying, "I just got a mental picture that might have some meaning for you. I saw a young boy flying down the street on a red bicycle, and he seems very happy, but I feel very sad."

The counselor said to me, "So do I," and tears began to run down his face. He said, "I was ten years old and that was my first bicycle. And it was the last time I remember ever feeling free or happy." He added, "I could ride the bicycle and I felt so free and alive. Then my father insisted I attend a university even though I hated it, and take up a career like his. He encouraged me to marry a woman I did not love. I have not been happy since."

This man had known that he was not happy, but had not realized that he was carrying such tremendous resentment toward his father. The image of the bicycle enabled him to become aware, and to work on letting go of his resentment. He soon felt the kind of freedom he had experienced as a child, and was able to make many new choices for his life.

This experience highlights a number of important aspects of intuition. First, intuition enables a counselor to hear and sense things which a client is experiencing but may not be able to put into words, or which the client may not even be aware of at the moment. Secondly, it is important for the counselor to be aware of the way in which his or her intuition speaks. For some, it is as though a light goes on in the mind, and they simply *know* something to be true.

For others, intuition speaks as a feeling or hunch. They may have a strong sense of an event that is going to take place, or of an action they must avoid. We have all heard of people who had strong premonitions about getting on an airplane that later crashed. Still other people, and I am one of them, find their intuition speaking most clearly by way of mental images or pictures. It is important to refrain

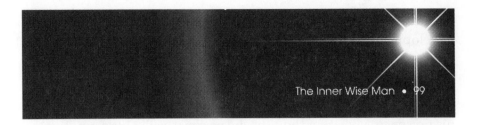

from making judgments about the value or meaning of an intuition.

Lack of trust in our innate intuitive ability is the first obstacle we face. We all have the gift of intuition, just as we have the ability to think and to reason and to imagine. Unfortunately, for most of us this ability is in a latent or dormant state. It needs to be actualized and released in order to assist us. Our ability has to be trained and disciplined until it becomes an art form that is second nature, such as singing or painting. It takes work and practice and patience, but first we must believe we have the ability.

As a young man, on my first trip to Hawaii, some local Hawaiians invited me to try using a surfboard. I told them I would like to learn, but even as a very young boy I had not been well-coordinated. It took me longer than others to learn things which required balance, like skating or riding a bicycle. I now know that I do not suffer from poor muscle coordination. Some forgotten adult had told me that and I believed it.

The Hawaiians said to me, "Do you really want to learn to surf?" I said, "Yes, but I am not very well coordinated." They laughed and said, "Well, that's all right, we will teach you." So I began my lessons. I fell off the board many times, but they would make a joke out of it. I would laugh with them, get back on the board and try again. Instead of work, it was like a game, with much playfulness and laughter. Soon I relaxed—and that was the key. One day I stood on the board and I *knew*. I knew the feeling of balance. I will never forget the joy of riding that first wave all the way to the shore. The Hawaiians jumped from their boards and came running to the shore to embrace me and congratulate me.

Our own negative, critical mind can be the greatest obstacle to developing our intuition. As a child I believed that I was not intuitive. I had a sister who was very intuitive. Even as a little girl, she told my father that a business associate was not trustworthy; she did not want to be in the same room with him because she felt so uncomfortable in his presence. My father thought she was just a silly little girl. But the man was not honest and my father lost about ten thousand dollars in an investment with this person. At that time I felt that my sister had a special gift which I did not have. It was not until I attended some workshops to train my intuition that I came to realize I possess a very good, functioning intuition.

I had an interesting experience in my first workshop on intuition. The leader was a very gifted intuitive woman who instructed us to report any impression which came to us about anyone in the workshop. At one point, early in the workshop, I approached her during a coffee break and said to her, "I have a strong impression about you." She invited me to share it with her. I said, "Does the name 'Martinez' have some special connection with you?" She replied, "No, I am sorry, but it does not." And I thought to myself, "You see, you are not intuitive at all. This proves it." My critical attitude was very active at that time!

Then the leader asked me, "What does the name 'Martinez' mean to you?" I said, "It is the name of someone from Mexico." The woman smiled and said, "Well, you are on target. I was born in Mexico City, of Mexican parents." Nothing about this woman's physical appearance or her speech patterns indicated that she might be Mexican. European, French or German perhaps, but not Mexican. I began to suspect that my intuition might just possibly be starting to function. Later we were asked to move into a meditative state and respond to different people in the group. I found that my impressions or images were very accurate. I came to believe in the power of my intuition as a result of these experiences.

Robert Ornstein has helped us to understand the functioning of

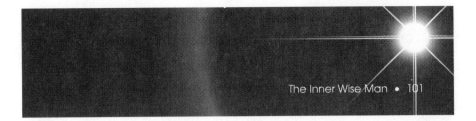

the mind by explaining the specialization of the two hemispheres of the brain. The left brain functions like a computer. It processes information, analyzes, makes judgments, and represents the rational part of the mind. It is very valuable, but unfortunately it does not produce any new information. The right brain provides that. It is the source of our imagination, intuition and creativity, and gives us new perspectives, new alternatives and new focus.

The tendency in our culture and in our educational system is to emphasize the use and training of the left brain and to ignore the right brain; thus as we grow to adulthood we are rather handicapped mentally. We have great ability at analysis and critical judgment, but very little ability in the area of imagination and creative alternatives. And our intuition is similarly weak.

In addition, Ornstein pointed out that the right and left brain hemispheres do not function well simultaneously. They work in much the same way as a television set; you cannot watch channel one and channel two at the same time. If we are "tuned in" to the left brain by our critical judgments, or if we are constantly trying to solve our problems by analyzing them, we remain stuck in that channel. In order to see a new perspective or focus, or a new possibility, we need to switch channels. We can do this by quieting the action of the left brain through body relaxation, closing the eyes, and then turning on our imagination. Imagination is the key which opens the door to the right brain. As we see new images or pictures, our attention is focused on these rather than on our analysis or negative thoughts. Then, new experiences can occur, new perspectives can be seen, and our intuition can begin to function and communicate to us.

A few years ago I was in Germany conducting some workshops with German psychologists. At one point I was facilitating an encounter group of eight men and women. They had agreed to use English, because my knowledge of German is meager. For the first day they did speak in English, but by the second day they began to use German, especially when they were excited about something. I tried to follow their remarks, and occasionally asked the person sitting next to me to translate, but mostly I tried to listen with the heart rather than the head.

One woman in the group was asked why she was so silent, and she answered by saying, "Oh, it is because at this point in my life I really do not have any major problems. I am more interested in what the rest of you have to say. I do not have anything that I need to work on or to talk about."

As she spoke I had a very powerful reaction inside myself. It was as if I could feel her fear echoing in me, and it was very strong. However, I did not say anything to her at that moment. A few hours later, she did speak briefly in response to a remark of another group member, and as she spoke an image came into my mind. This time I said to her, "As you were speaking just now, I had a very unusual image appear in my mind. It may not have reference to you, but I would like to report it, if I may." The woman said, "Of course, please do tell me about it." I said to her, "I see very clearly a church, like a German cathedral, a very beautiful stone church with stained glass windows. I also see a woman dressed in black with a black veil over her hat, kneeling before the high altar. Behind her is a small casket, like that of a child, surrounded by candles. And as I see this my heart is filled with a great sadness."

The woman began to weep violently. She told me, "That was the church where I went to pray after I had an abortion. I was desolate. My lover rejected me, my father threw me out of the house, and I went to that church because it was the only place where I could find some solace."

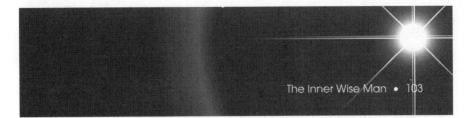

When she finished crying we did some Gestalt psychotherapy right there in the group. She was able to work through her feelings toward her father and her lover, to forgive them and herself, and to finish grieving for her dead child. In just one session she felt liberated and healed in her heart. This was a very powerful experience for everyone in that group. Some of the members were astonished by what they thought was a special psychic gift which I possessed. They were even more surprised to learn that it was more a matter of developing this gift than being born with highly actualized psychic powers. They were also encouraged to discover that they too could develop their intuition and learn to use it effectively as an aid to their psychotherapy and counseling.

Intuition permits a counselor to help clients become aware of aspects of their experience that are just as important as this woman's losses were to her, even though they may be less dramatic. I recall one therapist who came to me for counseling very concerned about a deteriorating relationship with his son. They argued constantly, the son was angry and rebellious, and the father felt very frustrated and helpless.

As the father was speaking I had an image of him in a sailboat on the open sea. When I reported my image to him, he laughed and said, "You know, that is what I would love to be doing. I would love to take some time off from work and sail on my boat. I am overstressed and I need to learn how to relax and how to play again. In fact, I really do not want to talk about my problem with my son. I want to talk about my problem with myself, and some decisions I have to make at this point in my life." Until presented with the image of the sailboat, this man was under the impression that the principal obstacle to his growth and inner peace was his son. The sailboat stimulated an awareness that he was really concerned with improving the quality of his life. Intuitive images can sow the seeds of new growth and personal change.

The benefits of having a healthy, functioning intuition are many and varied. Besides its value in counseling, I have discovered that new dimensions of experience become available to us. Life becomes richer and fuller, and rightly so, for we are functioning more as whole persons, rather than being limited to our left brain activity.

Fortunately, intuition is gaining in respectability, and more people wish to activate their intuition. My own experience suggests that people can achieve this goal best in the context of a group workshop. However, it is also possible to do it by ourselves by means of books or tapes now available.

For those interested in experimenting by themselves, let me share a fairly simple process which I have found most helpful. The first step is to relax the body by deep breathing, and sometimes by some kind of body movement. Exercises which increase tension in the muscles and then release that tension are helpful. Slow, deep breathing is important to facilitate the relaxation of the body.

The second step is to close the eyes and imagine a scene of nature: a lake, a river, mountains, a meadow—anything which is beautiful and restful. The purpose of this is to quiet the left brain activity and "switch channels" so that intuition can function. It is important to use the senses to enjoy the scene and to *experience* it rather than just to *think about* it.

The third step is to remain in the place of beauty, enjoying it, while allowing yourself to move gently into another, deeper level of consciousness. As this takes place, some kind of impression will come to you. It may be a feeling or it may be an image. The important thing to remember is that you do not *try* to bring about this impression. Nor do you allow the left brain to suggest doubts or

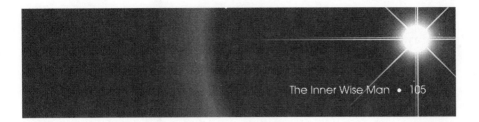

anxieties about the emergence of the impression. You focus on the scene and its beauty, and *allow* images or feelings to emerge. Trying to make intuition work is self-defeating.

Intuition is like a little child. It responds well to playful invitation but not to commands. It delights in fun but not in work. If you say to a child, "You must wash your face," the child is most likely to say, "No!" However, if you say to the child, "Let's see who can wash the quickest," the child is more likely to accept the challenge of a game. So, it is better not to try and force the mind, or to worry about being successful. Gradually, an intuitive sensing will emerge and grow stronger.

These, then, are simple steps toward activating our intuition. If you have a particular decision that you want to make, or need information about a person or situation, simply formulate a brief expression of your intention, repeat it several times to yourself, and then allow it to become a part of your stored information. This intention will be operating as you activate your intuition.

Perhaps the fastest way to activate intuition is to exercise it with another person who is also interested in developing his or her intuitive powers. The sharing and support seem to make the process work much better and also much quicker. I have found that, in the beginning, it is important for a person to spend at least fifteen minutes a day doing the nature fantasy. This teaches us to relax quickly and to move into another level of consciousness easily and naturally.

A side-effect reported by many doing these exercises is a radical change in attitude. Negative feelings begin to disappear from their lives. They become more sensitive and open to other people and more aware of their changes in feelings, both physical and emotional.

Most people have little need for all the good advice offered by psychologists. They have their own inner wisdom. They do not need instruction, for they have their own inner teacher. Counselors' bright observations usually come from the head. Their clients have a greater need for wisdom that comes from the heart. They need loving listening. They need a compassionate appreciation of their pain and struggle. They need support and encouragement.

Intuition helps us to tune in to each others' hidden hungers and to offer the nourishment of our sensitive loving responses. It enables us to help our friends complete with greater ease and speed the difficult journey from fear to love.

# CHAPTER THIRTEEN

# *The Miracle of Waiting*

It was late afternoon. I watched the slanting rays of the sun filtering through the transparent autumn leaves of red and yellow, and I felt at peace. I was standing in a wooded area surrounding the famous golden pavilion in Kyoto, Japan. Sightseers, mostly Japanese, moved past me. Their sounds were softened by dense moss and fern foliage; they seemed very much a part of the peace-filled scene. Late afternoon in the fall is the perfect time to visit this famous shrine, for then the sun turns the gold leafed building the color of burnished apricot and deepens the color tones of cherry leaves and evergreens.

I sat on a stone bench and absorbed the beauty, slowly savoring the richness of it all. Gradually a sense of meaning began to gather and form within me: the mystery and wonder, the miracle, of waiting.

The golden pavilion, like a jewel in the priceless setting of nature, revealed to me the source of this mystery. At one time its purpose was functional: housing people and ritual ceremonies. Now its purpose seems to be simply that of sharing its incredible beauty with others. To do this, the pavilion with its lovely surrounding wooded park must wait, wait for people to come and see, to taste and enjoy, and be nourished by its beauty.

This insight was the beginning of a series of reflections on the theme of waiting. The result was a radically different way of looking at this inevitable element of human life. Something in me was touched as I sat in that park in Kyoto that has enabled me to see waiting in a new, creative way.

Some of this change stems from my love of autumn. Autumn, for me, has always been a lovely, long, lingering season. It speaks to me of nature in a stage of waiting. Autumn comes after the passion of summer and before the freeze of winter. It lies somewhere between these two opposites, as a kind of bridge, and as a preparation, maintaining a foothold in the past as well as a contact with the future. I see autumn as a gift that allows us time to pause and reflect, to extend our experience of enjoyment in the present as we wait in expectation for the future. In autumn I am reminded that things, and people, must die, but that each death is also a beginning of new life. I can see the process of waiting as an important part, an essential element, of that new life.

I like to be reminded of these things as autumn turns the maple leaves to orange, rust and pale gold. For then I begin to notice changes that speak to me more of life than of death. I see the evergreens putting forth new growth, and the squirrels gathering nuts for their winter meals. I see animals growing heavier pelts in preparation for the approaching cold. All these are signs of nature readying itself for the winter wait. Nature does not deny the fact of waiting, nor try to avoid it. Animals and growing things accept this process, and use it well.

How differently we humans handle the fact of waiting.

Generally, we tend to look upon waiting as an obstacle to our progress, or a nuisance. This means that we try to remove the obstacle or tolerate the nuisance. I know this has often been my approach to waiting in the past. Yet that afternoon by the golden pavilion I began to see and experience waiting in a new way.

Waiting seems to me to be a rare kind of miracle. It is an opportunity to slow down and relax as I prepare to move into the future. I find it easier to let go of the past, with its pain and resentments, to feel the reflected sun of compassion softening the edges of past disagreements or disappointments. I find it easier to look into the future with less anxiety and more confident expectancy. I am more inclined then to believe that whatever new beginnings are being readied for birth in my life will ultimately bear good fruit for me. Sometimes the harvest may be an experience of joy, or perhaps an enriching new lesson about life.

I suppose I could describe this as being *more patient* with the waiting process, but the word "patience" rings too dully in my ears. I feel much more active in the process than "patience" implies. It seems more like facing the future squarely and feeling good whatever the outcome. It means feeling comfortable with the realization that the oak truly is waiting within the planted acorn. It means seeing the waiting goodness in an event, or the beauty waiting to blossom in a person.

At the same time, the initial period of waiting may seem, as it does in nature, like a death. It may even feel like a death, with all the attendant pain that death implies. We may need another person to provide the touch of life that will turn the death-phase of waiting into the surging hope for new life. The story of Sleeping Beauty is really an allegory about waiting. The loveliness of the young maiden was in a state of apparently lifeless immobilization. In actuality she was in a state of waiting, waiting for the loving touch of a person who could bring her into a new life. And when she was touched by love, she arose from her death-sleep to begin a life in which she could share her beauty with others.

Many of us are similarly asleep, with the beauty of our selves, our talents and gifts immobilized. We too need the touch of a loving person to bring us to new life, so that others can share in our beauty. This miracle transforms waiting into a doorway, through which we may enter a new world of significance. Once this happens, we find it easier to appreciate the hidden beauty asleep in others.

To see waiting as a gift of time is to experience a whole new perspective on life. Fear can be transformed, pain can be borne, conflict can be transcended, if they are stepping-stones to the fullness of our true beauty. This perspective moves us from the darkness of negative emotions to the light of positive attitudes. Despair gives way to hope, and death gives way to life. Viktor Frankl illustrates this experience in his book, *Man's Search For Meaning*. This famous Jewish psychiatrist, while imprisoned in Auschwitz during World War II, tells of a moment when he was close to despair. As he looked out past the prison walls to the gray skies and the gray winter landscape, his soul was similarly dark.

But then his eye caught a light that was turned on in a distant farmhouse, and it illumined the sky near the house. Something stirred in Frankl's soul. He recalled the biblical phrase, "a light shone in the darkness," and to him, it was a symbol of hope, a light that had come into his life. Frankl began a new life in the prison camp, a life in which he shared the beauty of his hope and love with the other inmates, actualizing their own latent beauty and power to survive. What had seemed like death was, in reality, a miracle about to be born.

Today, when it seems so hard for us to stop our incessant rush of activity, we need a new vision and experience of waiting. Many of us are tired of doing. We yearn for the quiet nourishment of being. We even express it in subtle ways. We talk about "getting away" for a while, of slowing down, of looking into meditation. This is often a description of our hidden hunger for a new experience of inner beauty and inner peace.

I talked recently to a graduate student who has been a Navy pilot for a number of years and has had exciting adventures all over the world. He observed, "What I want to do at this point in my life is to plant some things and watch them grow." I think he summed it up for many of us. Life bears down on us; it seems to keep us going 'round and 'round, like hamsters in a cage. And what we want very much at times is to be able to stop the whirling, to get off the treadle; to listen and smell and taste and feel; to find new meaning for our lives. Waiting can provide this kind of meaning for us.

The miracle of waiting is the miracle of life out of death, the wonder of emergence from apparent dead ends. When we share in this miracle, we are willing to allow time for seeds to grow and fruit to ripen. We have peace during this dormant period because we know that "for everything there is a season"; a time to laugh, a time to cry, a time to be born, and a time to die.

Shortly after I visited the shrine of the golden pavilion in Kyoto, I came across a passage by a Buddhist writer which describes a person who is aptly called the Awakened One: "I bide my time, a servant waiting for his wages. It is not death, it is not life I cherish. I bide my time in mindfulness and wisdom steeped."

This is the miracle of waiting: knowing deep within oneself that the future which emerges from this active waiting will be rich with meaning. I need not cling to the past nor yearn for the future. I need merely open myself to the present, awaiting with confident expectancy the new directions that will bring new life and inner peace.

## CHAPTER FOURTEEN

# *Specialness, the Key to Self-Esteem*

I can recall the scene clearly. It is mid-afternoon in a hillside suburb of Los Angeles. The sun is edging toward the western horizon and a warm breeze whips my hair as I race home from school. Nearing the house I can smell it: freshly baked bread! As I dash through the kitchen door I am greeted with a hug from my grandmother and then taken to the breakfast room. There, at the head of the table, I find my treasure: a small, individually baked cinnamon-and-sugar-topped coffee cake.

The significance is not lost on me as I munch the still-warm cake and wash it down with a glass of cold milk. This is not a piece from the larger cake baked for the family. This was made specially for me and served to me at the head of the table. Once again I am reminded that, in the eyes of my grandmother, I am a very special person. To this day, whenever I smell the aroma of baking bread I remember that scene and think with gratitude of the woman who made me feel so loved.

I contrast this with the experiences of a group of recovering drug addicts who recalled their childhoods with anger and bitterness. Far from having felt special, they had felt unloved and unwanted. Struggling to build their sense of self-esteem from the ashes of these tragic beginnings, they found it difficult to have faith in themselves and trust in others. Without trust they were not able to enjoy loving relationships, which left them with deep feelings of loneliness. G. B. Stern speaks of this as, "the terrible feeling of not being first with anyone." Unfortunately, their loneliness will most likely continue until they find someone with a love great enough to tolerate their self-destructive anger; great enough to overcome their self-hatred; someone who believes in them even when they cannot believe in themselves.

Some years ago a noted priest and author described his experience with such a person. He told of being invited to lunch with a former high school student. Over hamburgers, the young man, then about to graduate from college said, "Father I wanted to meet with you to thank you for what you have given me. For tour years you put up with me acting like an idiot, testing you, rebelling against everything you stood for, and yet whenever I needed you, you were there for me. Somehow you made me feel special. You believed in me when I didn't believe in myself. Well, I am beginning to believe in myself, and it's only because of your love that never failed me." My priest friend said that not only was he amazed by this expression of gratitude, but that it changed his entire approach to teaching. He began to listen more carefully to the inner needs of his students and was better able to offer them the kind of caring that enabled them to appreciate *their own individual specialness.*

Looking back on my own experience of school, I can recall a few teachers who, in small ways, helped me to become aware of and to actualize some of my special, but latent, talents. I remember a nun who chided me for not expanding my intellectual interests. She opened up the new worlds of science and literature to me and fostered an interest in writing. I am also grateful for a high school drama teacher who talked me out of my self-doubts and into a play where I stole the show. And I can never forget the librarian, a brilliant woman with two doctorates, who debated ideas with me as if I were her equal. With her I always felt respected and valued as a special friend.

Each of these persons gave me something of themselves that made it possible for me to discover a hidden part of myself. Our growth in self-esteem begins in these relationships, in which others see something in us that we have not been able to see. We are built up by their faith in us even when we are unable to believe in ourselves.

Self-esteem blossoms through this process of uncovering and discovering. With loving support and encouragement, we are able to take the risk of pulling back our self-protective curtain—and suddenly we become aware of a new section of the mosaic of our inner beauty. At the same time, we must be willing to change our self-perception, to release the fixed image of ourselves that we have maintained.

Letting go is easier when we realize that our old image is partial and thus distorted, like the image we see in amusement park mirrors. If we would see our true selves, we need to look into the eyes of people who love us, for they reflect our true beauty. And once we perceive this beauty, latent talents and abilities can come alive, nourished by our new sense of inner worth and personal power. Norman Cousins, writing of Albert Schweitzer, said, "Each man has his own potential in terms of achievement and service. The awareness of the potential is the discovery of purpose, the fulfillment of that potential is the discovery of strength."

Fostering the discovery by another person of their specialness can be a test of the genuineness of our love. Often our loving consists in *doing for* others. But this may well rob them of the joy of discovering for themselves. A more difficult gesture—but more genuinely loving—is that of offering our companionship and encouragement to the person setting out on the road to self-discovery, and sharing their delight in reaching the end of the journey.

Virginia Satir, the pioneer of family therapy, was able to give this kind of love generously and artfully in her workshops. I recall one occasion on which she invited a participant to join her in front of a large group and share his insights about a previous exercise. With genuine warmth, Virginia put her arm around the shoulders of this young man, who was obviously nervous. She asked him to tell her something about himself, and as he relaxed he began to discuss what he had learned.

Then Virginia did a wonderful thing. Very gently she interrupted him, and turning to the audience she pointed out how his comments illustrated principles she had stressed in her lecture. She did this several times, deepening and expanding the insights, so that the young man suddenly became aware of the richness of his remarks. With Virginia's help he not only felt respected; he also discovered a new way to work with an insight, to play with it, allow it to grow and bear new fruit. In thanking Virginia he said that this awareness was like finding a new treasure within himself. And it happened because Virginia, like all great teachers and true lovers, knew the importance of resisting the temptation to simply give a gift. She preferred to join the person in the search for the treasure.

Anyone who has taught or counseled can testify to the fact that we are surrounded by people of all ages and backgrounds who need to discover their specialness, whose self-esteem is at the poverty level. But how can we recognize them, since most of them have learned to hide their feelings of inadequacy and hurt? There is one way that is foolproof: to look at them with the eyes of the heart rather than through the microscope of our value judgments. Saint-Exupery has expressed it well: "It is only with the heart that one can see rightly; what is essential is invisible to the eye."

As self-esteem begins to grow we must learn to be patient. It is like a lovely plant that grows slowly. It has to be fed regularly with small amounts of nourishment, and it must be placed in an environment suited to its unique needs. Short-term lovers often are more interested in the fruits of their love than in the well-being of the loved one. Like impatient gardeners, they want to force the plant to bloom quickly. Genuine lovers are more willing to continue their caring and support even when they do not see immediate results.

Faith is confirmed when the loved one translates new feelings of self-worth into actions which result in small successes. Old feelings of inadequacy give way to new feelings of self-confidence. An actor once told me, "I will never forget my first stage success. Some hidden power seemed to take over, and as I made my exit I heard this thunderous applause. They were applauding little old me! I had stopped the show. My self-esteem took on new meaning as I realized the kind of power I possess to move an audience."

Success experiences such as this one give new depth to our sense of specialness because they demand new risks. Not only do we have to step into a new arena of fear, but we have to face this challenge alone. Support may be present, but it is waiting in the wings. When we overcome the fear and accomplish the task, we have the added reward of being able to say, "I did it. No one else did it for me." This is the moment when we discover not only our inner beauty but also our inner strength.

It is equally important that we do not dismiss the fact that *all personal growth involves some pain*. There is no quick and painless way. By its nature, growth demands death, a process of undoing, before new life-forms can be created. We may be tempted to try and avoid the pain or to escape the hurt. But that is when loving friends can be a priceless resource. They remind us that the pain is both necessary and bearable. They can be with us in our pain, helping us to accept it and even to appreciate its importance in our growth process. Bernie Siegel reminds us that humor may also place pain in its proper perspective. In his book, *Love, Medicine and Miracles* he tells of finding the garbage disposal in his home jammed. He asked his wife, "What shall I do?" His wife replied, "Just push the reset button." And Bernie then addressed a silent question to God, "Why didn't you give us a reset button?" The reply that came to him was very telling, "I did, Bernie. It's called pain and suffering." Perhaps that is why Indian writers refer to pain as "a cosmic necessity."

There is a marvelous paradox about helping others to discover their specialness. An Eastern story tells of a man who is taken on a visit to both hell and heaven. In hell he sees a group of people around a table laden with all kinds of delicacies. But they are emaciated and starving. Looking more carefully, the visitor sees that they have been given chopsticks that are extremely long. Although they can pick up the food, when they try to bring it to their mouths, the chopsticks carry it past their mouths and over their shoulders, and it is lost.

In heaven, the visitor sees a similar table—but here the people are fat and smiling. His guide explains that although their chopsticks are similarly long, the people in heaven have discovered the secret of life, which is love. They have discovered that in feeding others first, they in turn are fed.

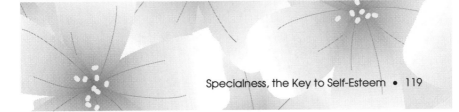

This is the lovely paradox for lovers who foster the discovery of specialness in others. In reaching out to others, they themselves are touched. When they allow others to see love mirrored in their eyes, they find that love reflected in the eyes of the loved one. The truth of the prayer of Saint Francis has become for them an existential reality: "It is in giving that we receive."

CHAPTER FIFTEEN

# *When You Hear the Music*

Picture this scene: a television talk show. A smiling host is listening to his beautiful celebrity guest describe her latest film. Suddenly, music is heard in the background. The actress hears it, but is intent on making one final comment about her film and continues to talk. As a result, television viewers see her being cut off in mid-sentence as they are switched to a commercial featuring a pair of dentures in a bubbly liquid.

A rare occurrence? Not as rare as television producers would want. And what does it mean? To me, it is an excellent example of the fact that when we have a personal investment in an issue, we do not listen very well. We hear things, but fail to pay attention to, or often ignore, what we hear. This is especially true for things that are unpleasant or frightening.

Such selective inattentiveness may reflect old patterns for us. Freud would probably trace it back to our early childhood, when we learned to tune out demands and scoldings from parents:

"Billy, ARE YOU LISTENING TO ME?"

"Uh-huh."

Whatever its cause, the effects can range from mischief-making in relationships to personal disaster. Lawrence LeShan, Ph.D. discovered that sixty-eight out of seventy terminally-ill patients he studied reported feeling severe depression prior to the onset of their illness. The warning signs were present, the background music was playing, but these people chose to ignore or deny the alarms. Like these terminal patients, we too may be failing to heed the warning signs that come from our overstressed bodies. In my case, I tend to ignore the indications that I am overly tired. I push and prod my body until it simply rebels, and I am forced to rest by reason of a bad cold or flu.

More challenging than attending to the messages sent by our bodies is the ability to note changes in our moods or emotions. These are much subtler and more easily recognized in hindsight. A group of women interviewed on a television panel concerning the infidelity of their husbands admitted that, in looking back, they were able to recall mood swings and sudden bursts of emotion in their husbands. Some of these men switched from being easygoing to being irritable. Others moved from being gentle to being angry, or from being accepting to being demanding. None of the women recognized these changes as alerting signals that something was wrong. The lesson they learned, which is equally important for us, is that any sudden change in mood or emotion speaks of powerful inner stirrings. It cannot be ignored without paying a price, often a very painful one.

Knowing our weak spots can enable us to recognize the danger signs sooner. A friend of mine told me, "I have two indications that

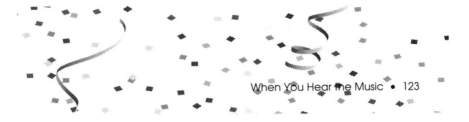

I am overstressed. One is a grouchy mood in which I am irritable with everyone and everything. The other is a state of being very defensive and clinging to my opinions as if they were infallible." I asked this man how he responds after he becomes aware of these alerts. He said, "I take time out. I might have a hot beverage with a friend, I may have a nap or take a walk in the fresh air, I may do a little painting. But the main thing is that I am allowing my body and mind to release some of the stress." His response is a wise one. Rather than deny or ignore the presence of stress, he faces it and accepts the challenge of doing something about it.

The Senoi tribe in Malaysia have a wonderful way of teaching this lesson to their children. Each morning the family members share their dreams, and the parents use these as opportunities to impart essential values to their youngsters. They tell the story of a young boy who described his dream. "Last night I dreamed of a tiger," he said.

The parents asked, "What happened?"

The boy replied, "The tiger was very big and I was very frightened, so I ran away, and then I woke up." Then the parents imparted their lesson: "Ah, that was because you do not understand about dream-tigers. The tigers you meet during the day can harm you and so it is wise to run from them. But the tigers in your dreams have no power to harm you unless you give them that power. So, the next time you dream of a tiger, instead of running away, *turn and face the tiger!*"

The following week the boy excitedly reported, "I dreamed of a tiger again, and I did what you said, and do you know what happened? The tiger ran away!" This fortunate child was learning at an early age that a person is better served by facing reality rather than trying to escape from it. He also learned that facing a fearful challenge mobilizes latent sources of energy and courage.

Elisabeth Kubler-Ross has traced for us the various stages of dying. She has pointed out that during the early stages, people use denial, anger and bargaining as ways of trying to avoid or escape the brutal facts. Then finally truth dawns, at which point the dying person often feels helpless and becomes depressed and despairing. It seems that all is lost. And yet, out of the seed-bed of this despair, there often comes the tiny shoot of new life, of a spirit reborn. It is only then, when the facts have been faced and reality accepted, that a great inner peace can follow.

Norman Cousins and Dr. Carl Simonton have also attested to the fact that terminal patients who abandon attitudes of denial are able to energize their healing powers in a dramatic way. Many cancer patients they interviewed experienced complete remission after they "faced the tiger" and chose to engage in a fight for their lives. Their initial assumption that the word "terminal" was an irreversible death sentence began to change. They felt a renewed desire to live and an enkindled faith in their ability to heal their bodies.

The mere fact that we experience something tragic or traumatic *does not necessarily mean that our lives will be affected in a permanently negative manner.* As many of us have learned, some of these painful moments can be blessings in disguise. An automobile accident, the birth of a deformed child, the sudden loss of a loved one, a serious illness—these can act as thunderbolts to our beliefs and value systems, jolting us into transformative action. They can force us to re-evaluate our lives, to make important changes in our behavior and lifestyle.

Steven McAuliffe, whose wife Christa perished in the NASA Challenger disaster, is a man whose life has been altered dramatically. In a recent interview he said, "I have a recognition that my days are few and I'm going to do some of the things I always wanted to do." His response to tragedy is an example of what some writers term "seizing the moment."

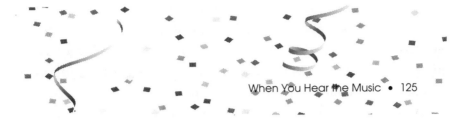

This urgency to act rather than talk or ponder, to respond now rather than later, can set us upon a new path and radically change our lives. The initial action could be as simple as making a phone call that brings us to a group of supportive people. Or it could be as challenging as forgiving someone who has hurt us.

A client once shared with me the results of this kind of choice for him. His relationship with his father had been poor. He resented the fact that his father had not spent much time with him as a child and seemed incapable of expressing affection. A serious illness prompted the son to go to his father and tell him of his love. He said to his father, "I realize now that you were not able to show your love for me in the way I wanted it shown. But I also know that you loved me deeply and in the best way you knew how. I'm sorry for holding resentment toward you and want you to forgive me because I love you very much." His father didn't say a word at first. Then his eyes filled with tears and he embraced his son. Only then could he say to his son, "This is one of the happiest moments of my life. I was never able to be expressive like your mother. I just hoped that somehow you would know I loved you by the things I did for you. Now I know."

The choice to seize the moment not only moves us in new ways. It keeps us moving by focusing our attention on the immediate action and the next few steps to be taken. We do not waste energy speculating about the distant goal. This approach moves us past the blockade of denial, guides us through the minefields of fear, and carries us beyond the paralysis of victimhood. With each small step on the new path we find our confidence and courage growing. The formerly powerful voice inside us, always telling us to BEWARE! is gradually replaced by a gentler, reassuring voice, reminding us to BE AWARE!

Sensitive listening to the "background music" coupled with a prompt response are difficult skills, but ones which can be learned. We acquire them best by being with people who are good models for us: a caring friend whom we trust, a skillful therapist, a supportive group. These people enable us to detect the warning signs sooner. They encourage us as we struggle to respond to the challenge of change.

Recently, a University of Hawaii cheerleader discovered the value of this kind of support. Severely injured during a team practice, she was told that she might not walk again. She faced the reality of her injury, but not the verdict. She chose to mobilize her inner resources, believing she could find a way to walk anew. Not only her classmates, but the entire community rallied to help her through the long months of therapy on her damaged nerves and muscles.

Then it happened. One evening during half-time of a football game, aided only by a walker, this brave young woman made her slow journey to the center of the field. The crowd of thousands, silent at first, rose to their feet and cheered. She was deluged with flower leis. It was a night of great achievement, of tears and joy, and of sharing the love that had made her success possible.

Success in any aspect of living is determined by our response when we hear the music start to play in the background. In order to achieve our goals and realize our dreams, we must learn to pay attention not only to the world around us, but also to the messages we receive from our bodies and our inner emotions. As we begin to pay attention, to notice, all of our senses become sharper. Like a patient after a cataract operation, things jump out at us—things always present but never really noticed before. Our intuition, especially, becomes more available and more reliable, and our willingness to take risks begins to grow.

What then should we do when we hear the music? We should stop talking and start listening. We should open our inner ears to the message behind the sounds, to the meaning and purpose of the signs demanding our attention. Next, we should seize the moment and act.

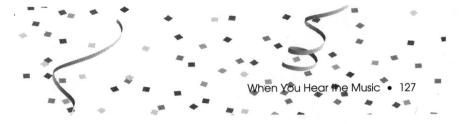

These two steps will bring us into a new experience of inner power and give us a sense of direction in our lives.

Corita Kent, the late serigraph artist, sums up the heart of this approach in one of her famous posters. In it she says, "Life is a series of moments. To live each one is to succeed."

# CHAPTER SIXTEEN

# *The Illusion Trap*

We all have our moments of craziness. To be human means to be a little crazy occasionally. The kind of craziness that we want to avoid is the *patterned thinking* which causes us to confuse reality with unreality. I am referring to attitudes and expectations which are based on myths or illusions. These are subtly erosive of our mental health and can become traps from which it is difficult to extricate ourselves.

Every illusion or false belief has the appearance of truth. If this were not the case, magicians would have ceased to delight their audiences with tricks of rabbits and vanishing scarves. Appearances can be deceptive, and expectations can prompt us to believe we see things which in reality we do not see. This may begin in childhood, which is essentially a time of budding faith. As children, we believe what our parents tell us about ourselves and our small world. They convince us that we are lovable or we are clumsy; that Santa Claus brings toys to good children; that if we are hurt, Mother will kiss us and make us well; that if a toy is broken, Daddy can fix it.

Contained in these childhood expressions of faith is a hidden assumption that *responsibility for our lives and happiness rests in the hands of others.* Later, as adults, we will search for a man or woman to complete our lives, little realizing that we may still be bound by the same illusion. We may be putting the responsibility for our happiness upon the shoulders of our partners, not realizing that the attainment of our dreams is primarily the product of our own actions.

This kind of thinking is crazy-making. We are diminished and weakened by it. Placing responsibility for our lives in the hands of others leaves us helpless, makes us feel like victims—devoid of energy and, above all, hope. Awareness of this perverse pattern can restore us to vibrant emotional health and awaken a sense of inner power. Recently a client said to me, "I just realized that I have been a 'good girl' for twenty-five years, trying to please everyone. Well, I don't need that any more. I don't need to please my parents and I don't need to beg for approval from my husband. From now on I'm giving myself permission to do what I think is right for me. And you know, it feels great!" Abandoning the myth that transforming power had to come from an outside source, this woman discovered new sources of inner power and hope. She gained release from her personal illusion trap.

A similar discovery is described in *The Wizard of Oz.* Dorothy and her three companions sought out the Wizard because they believed he had the magic needed to solve their problems. This myth was first dented when the Wizard said they would have to kill the Wicked Witch before their wishes would be granted. They discovered that they had to work for their magic rather than receive it as a free gift from the Wizard.

As the story unfolds we see the Wizard's wisdom. The problems of Dorothy and her companions had a common root: a feeling of powerlessness. The Wizard could have told them they already possessed the power to change their lives. Instead he chose to let each one discover this truth through personal experience.

Upon the completion of their mission, the Tin Woodman found that he did possess a heart, full of compassion and tenderness. The Scarecrow discovered that he had a fine mind and was able to think clearly and creatively. The Cowardly Lion found that he could function despite his fears. And Dorothy realized that she had only to click her slippers together in order to be transported wherever she wished. How wonderful that these four individuals were able to change themselves from helpless victims to peak performers. At the same time, how sad that they had existed in the prison of their own illusions for so many years.

And how foolish, we might be tempted to think. Yet, abandoning self-defeating beliefs is not as easy as it may seem. Even when we are informed of these patterns, we find it difficult to let go of them. W. H. Auden said:

> We would be rather ruined than changed
> We would rather die in our dread
> Than climb the cross of the moment
> And let our illusions die.

At times we delude ourselves with the tenacity of a drowning person clinging to a log salvaged from the shipwreck of his life. I have heard a man declare, "I'm sure our marriage will improve after I retire." Perhaps it will, but most likely the marriage will experience greater stress, not less. I have also heard an abused child proclaim, "I swear I'll never treat my kids the way my parents treated me." I hope this will be the case, but research suggests that there is a greater likelihood he will become an abusing parent himself. In a similar manner, drug addicts and alcoholics profess beliefs which indicate to all except themselves the illusions which trap them. Only when they surrender these false beliefs can they find new power.

Letting go of these myths is somewhat easier when we recognize the arrogance they represent. We often assign divine infallibility to our illusory perceptions. Reality demands more humility from us. Few things in life are either black or white, totally right or absolutely wrong. The mosaic of life contains many different shapes and colors, and these can be interpreted differently as light and perspective affect our perceptions. Initial impressions can change with time and experience. Illusion is not so much a case of *untruth* as of *partial truth*. Humility asks that we grant ourselves the opportunity not to make rash judgments, but to examine things from a variety of viewpoints and be willing to alter our perceptions.

An example of the power of the altered perceptions can be seen in the field of preventive medicine. New horizons of healing are now appearing. The old belief, that the patient was a helpless victim awaiting the touch of a medical wizard, has changed. Today we are discovering ways in which we can promote healing within ourselves. We are learning new methods of mobilizing our inner resources of mind, body and spirit. We have a better sense of the relationship between our lifestyle and a healthy immune system. The benefits of this new knowledge are already evident in the treatment of life-threatening illnesses.

Transformation from helplessness to power begins with the

recognition that there are no wizards "out there." The magic of wizardry is within each of us. We all possess what we need for a healthy life and how to obtain it. All that is required for us to contact this inner source of wisdom is the willingness to be quiet, to listen meditatively. As we block out the sounds and sights of the world around us, we begin to enter into the world within us. Gradually we develop a clearer sense of things, an ability to separate truth from distortion, reality from illusion.

A new stage of transformation is attained when we learn to correct our course. No one grows by moving in a straight line. Our growth line usually looks like the path of a sailboat. We get off course and make adjustments to get back on course. We make errors and we correct them. And far from being discouraged by this method, we recognize it to be the slow, sure way to arrive at our destination. Illusion suggests we can do things perfectly the first time, that we can avoid mistakes. Humility tells us that much of our later wisdom will come to us not despite our errors, but because of them.

Finally, in the face of life's storms, whether these be minor showers or major hurricanes, we have choices. We can label these events as inevitable disasters or we can view them as challenges to immediate action. We can choose between sitting and soaring. By sitting, we prepare to be overwhelmed, to give in to our fate. By soaring, we mobilize our spirits to fly beyond the storm. Rather than giving in to our weaknesses, we choose to give them up.

Richard Bach has captured this passion to soar in his immensely popular book *Jonathan Livingston Seagull*. Like Jonathan, we find well-intentioned people with limited vision who look with scorn upon those of us who choose to risk, who expand our horizons. They label us "crazy" because we attempt things they deem impossible. But it is equally possible that, like Jonathan, we may discover that the real craziness is in believing we are victims rather than striving victors. Jonathan demonstrated that our spirits were made for soaring beyond our self-imposed barriers.

Soaring! How the very word causes our hearts to beat a little faster! It speaks to that part of us which will never die, which refuses to accept labels of doom and disaster, which seeks to develop our lives to their fullest dimensions. For some of us this spirit may have first caught fire when, as children, we were dazzled by the sight of kites sailing on a spring afternoon. For others it may have been a glimpse of birds, with brilliant flashes of color, flying towards the sun. For some of us, grown older, it can come alive in us as we see a jet plane silhouetted against a sunset sky. At such moments, something in us stirs, illusion fades away, and we *know*. We know we have a similar power, a divine gift enabling us to break free from present limitations, to go beyond our imagined barriers, to experience the joy of soaring.

We have the power. We need only be reminded of that fact. Jonathan's story remind us; the wonder of nature reminds us; during a meditative moment our inner healer reminds us. And for added encouragement we can take to heart the final lines of Dorothy's touching song from the movie version of *The Wizard of Oz:*

And the dreams that you dare to dream
Really do come true…
If happy little bluebirds fly
Beyond the rainbow,
Why oh why can't I?

# CHAPTER SEVENTEEN

# *A Matter of Focus*

Several years ago, while working with a school system, I gained an insight which has continued to be very valuable. As an organizational consultant it was my task to interview people from all sectors of the system. My findings uncovered the usual rivalries, power struggles, and breakdowns in communication. What surprised me was an almost universal sense of frustration and helplessness. I was surprised because the men and women I interviewed were intelligent and creative individuals. Yet somehow they had fine-tuned their focus exclusively to the negative aspects of their work environment. Their horizons were narrowed and their hopes were diminished by their chosen perspectives. It was evident that they could not have a happier work experience until they were willing to alter their negative focus.

With this in mind I scheduled a retreat for the top administrators at a beautiful, secluded mountain resort. For a day and a half the agenda was primarily directed towards relaxation and enjoyment. I invited the participants to set aside their problems temporarily, and to assist one another in the task of being nourished and relaxed by the beauty of nature and outdoor activities. Some took hikes or saunas together; others engaged in sports or swimming.

In the process of relaxing together these men and women discovered many things about one another that had been unknown previously. They shared common interests and family concerns. Many had similar hobbies. Talking about these things while sharing a lovely sunset or the tonic of sweet-smelling pines enabled them to meet one another as persons rather than as competitive colleagues.

Later, when we began our working sessions, the atmosphere was very different from previous staff sessions on campus. There was a general lightness of tone, a greater feeling of trust and openness. The mood seemed to have switched from a competitive to a cooperative one. The participants began to listen to each other in a new way. They became concerned about *the impact of problems on one another*, rather than focusing only on *the problems themselves*. Some of the old frustrations began to be replaced with confidence in their ability to join hands to create a safe path through the thorny issues they faced.

Several weeks after this retreat I joined them for a staff meeting on campus. I was delighted with the changes I observed. New lines of communication had been established between administrators and teachers. A consensus approach to decision-making had, after a clumsy start, become a satisfying and effective method for them. Opposing opinions and angry feelings could be heard and responded to—without defensiveness, in many instances. The teachers had also scheduled a series of pot-luck suppers where they could share good food and informal conversation, recapturing the substance of the retreat.

The net result of all these changes was a shift in focus. As they came to know and understand one another more personally, the teachers overcame previous fears and the need to protect themselves. Where they had once felt helpless in their separateness, they now felt powerful by reason of their sense of community. Most important, they were able to accomplish important projects because their creative energy was going into the discovery of new ways to attain their goals, rather than into fighting each other.

I have recalled that experience may times when faced with my own feelings of helplessness and frustration in the face of some challenge. It has made me more sensitive to clients struggling with similar feelings. These new, positive experiences enable clients to turn the prism of their focus from negative to positive. It reminds us both that beauty is found even in the darker blues and purples, as well as in the brighter yellow and oranges, of our experiential prisms.

The tragedy of a negative fixation is that it limits both our perspective of the present and the horizon of the future. When we choose to see only one aspect of a reality it is easy to become discouraged and despairing. A Vietnam veteran told me, "When I discovered that both my legs had been amputated, I could see myself in just one way, as a helpless cripple." Fortunately he met a caring nurse who was able to offer him a different way of viewing his situation. She said to him, "Your problem is that you are focusing on only one thing, what you have lost. What about those things you still possess: a basically strong body, a fine mind, and a great supply of untapped potential?" Gradually, he released his negative view and began to build his inner strength and his will to make a new, meaningful life for himself. Today he works with paraplegics, modeling the kind of change he challenges them to create for themselves. His reward is seeing other young men shift their perspectives and expand their horizons.

When feelings of gratitude are maintained, such transformations continue. Spiritual teachers have long insisted that forgiveness and gratitude are not only a path to inner peace but also a reward for the journey. Richard Bach suggests gaining perspective even at the onset of a negative experience. He says, "Every problem comes to us with a gift in its hand." Mother Teresa expressed the same feelings when a young woman was describing her personal problems in painful detail. This remarkable missionary said, "Problems! Problems! Everyone always refers to these things as problems. Is there not another word we can use? How about 'gift'?"

Altering our viewpoint is usually rather difficult, but it can be made easier by the support of caring people, and by the recognition that it is best accomplished in a series of small steps, rather than a miraculous flash of awareness. Keeping our attention on the next step rather than worrying about the length of the journey is a wise approach. Recovering alcoholics know this to be not only helpful but essential to their progress. Learning to live "one day at a time" enables us to keep our energy focused rather than allowing it to scatter into concern and anxiety.

Inner language also supports us in maintaining a new perspective. Listening to our inner monologue will quickly reveal a negative emphasis. We can then re-phrase our words to correct the imbalance. Instead of saying, "Oh, it is so difficult" we can state, "This is a difficult challenge, *and* I am going to find some creative alternatives." In place of saying, "I really don't know what to do," we can say, "I haven't found an answer *yet*, but I am determined to keep searching until I do." These slight changes in our speech are not merely prettier words, they tell the *whole* truth. They enable us to recognize the

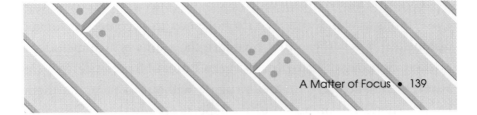

resources and options available as well as the difficulties.

Aikido similarly teaches its pupils a new consciousness concerning their energy. When attacked, they are taught to switch their focus from the attacker to the center of energy in their own bodies. They learn to maintain this positive focus by concentration. This delicate balance enables them to swiftly deflect blows from an attacker, and ultimately induce the opponent to lose his or her balance. By focusing on the positive energy rather than the dynamics of attack, they transform themselves from victims to persons who are in control of the situation.

One of the most striking examples of personal change by means of altered perspective is that of Helen Keller. Although deaf, dumb and blind as a child, she became a woman of outstanding accomplishment. With the loving assistance of Annie Sullivan, Helen was able, by very gradual steps, to change her initial cry of "I can't" to a triumphant, "I can!" Despite her handicaps, Helen expanded her horizons to include lecture platforms and friendships with people all over the world.

Everyone has his or her limitations and imperfections. That is a given. The good news is that they do not have to be permanent obstacles in our growth. We can *choose* not to be limited by our limitations. Ernest Holmes has said, "It is possible to get sugar even from a cracked sugar bowl." We can elect to focus on what we possess rather than on what we do not have. What matters most is not the perfection of our inner sugar bowls, but the value and worth of the contents. We can contact and experience our inner goodness by the simple, though at times difficult and challenging, process of transforming our negative fixation.

This is a matter of focus. We do not have to pretend that everything is wonderful. We do not need to become "cock-eyed optimists." It is sufficient that we face the reality which includes a positive and negative aspect to every human experience. We can admit the challenge, pain and struggle without focusing on them. Every experience contains positive aspects of growth, new learning, awakened consciousness and a change of priorities. We need not put on rose colored glasses. We need only remove our dark glasses and open our eyes to the beauty around and within us.

Transformation is very much like opening our eyes to the glory of the rainbow, which occurs only when there is also a storm or falling rain. If we are especially blessed we will find loving friends to share the joy of the rainbow, people with whom we exchange delight and laughter at the wonder of such blazing beauty in our lives.

CHAPTER EIGHTEEN

# *The Other Side of Failure*

"Failure" can be a tough label to remove. Like those adhesive price stickers which resist fingernails and hot water, the label of failure tends to cling to our actions and our sense of self worth. Perhaps we need to re-examine our concept of failure, and to inspect the other side of the coin.

Our culture has a narrow notion of failure. Limited by our dualistic thinking, we tend to view it primarily as the opposite of success. And since success is the ultimate achievement, failure becomes the ultimate disaster.

Eastern thinking sees failure as a part of life's ongoing pattern of learning and growing. In that view, life is comprised of negative and unpleasant elements as well as of positive and pleasant ones. The Eastern philosopher does not consider these to have moral connotations of good and bad. Success and failure are joined together, like male and female, and from this union comes new life in the form of knowledge and experience.

There is a hint of this concept in one sector of our culture, the scientific community. Scientific researchers view failure as an essential part of the process of data acquisition. Every experiment has the potential for providing new information, valuable in the structuring of future experiments. Breakthroughs are achieved most often as a result of a series of failures. From each failed experiment comes the knowledge of what does not work, accompanied by the challenge to seek alternative approaches.

We can expand our own personal understanding of failure by unmasking some long-held myths. One of these is the connection between failure and discouragement. We often feel that because we have failed in one instance we should stop striving. Another myth sees failure as a permanent disaster or ultimate defeat, rather than a temporary setback containing the opportunity to take a new direction.

Many people with celebrated careers discovered their unique talents only through experiences with failure. Elsie de Wolfe, the woman who created the concept of interior design and decoration, struggled for years to become an actress, without any significant success. Audiences seemed to be more interested in her fashionable clothes than in her performances on stage. Her plays were mostly dramatic failures. Elsie eventually realized that she could create a different kind of drama with clothes, and later with the interiors of homes. It was her failure as an actress that led her into a career that made her a celebrity in Europe and America, as well as a very wealthy woman.

Jean Piaget also found his life taking a new direction as a result of his experiences with failure. While testing the intelligence of children, he became fascinated with the failures of the children, with

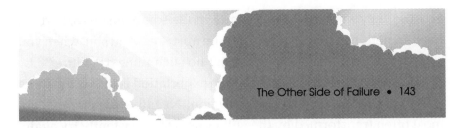

their *wrong* answers. Pursuing these, he discovered the ways in which a child's mind develops, which led to his famous theory of cognitive development. Today, millions of teachers have been aided and influenced by Piaget's writings.

These examples remind us that the myth of failure can mask opportunities hidden in our disappointing experiences. A sudden illness or accident, a radical change in lifestyle, or the loss of someone dear to us can trigger a change in our view of failure. Viktor Frankl discovered this among his fellow prisoners in Auschwitz. Uprooted from everything which had spelled success and security, they fell into a terrible depression at first.

As their will to survive grew their priorities changed. They saw their current experience as a challenge to stop focusing on hate and start focusing on love. They sought to improve the quality of the life they had together. Food, bits of soap and thread, gifts of poetry and art were shared. Men too ill to work were replaced by those who were stronger. Feelings of failure disappeared and feelings of satisfaction and achievement replaced them. Even in the face of death these men and women experienced a kind of loving community that surpassed any they had known before.

One of the obvious lessons from the Auschwitz experience is the power of shared love. It is not easy to alter our perspective of failure, but it becomes easier when we have loving people who support us and assist us in discovering ways to redefine failure and success. Even a humorous remark, given with care, can make it possible for us to see failure in a different light. A Midwestern farmer is reputed to have said to his grandson, "Son, they put erasers on pencils because they know we are going to make some mistakes, and we need something handy to correct those mistakes. And son, when you can correct your mistakes, there ain't no such thing as failure."

The fear of not living up to some expectation is overcome more effectively by action than by reflection. Negative experiences are most often transformed by the willingness to persistently try again. Moshe Feldenkrais, a great teacher of body therapists, put heavy emphasis on the value of repeated efforts. He would tell his students, "your body can re-learn anything it needs to re-learn." He developed a series of repeated exercises through which the body could release tension and enhance muscular ability. Some of his students had lived for years with crippling forms of illness, yet were able to overcome their severe physical restrictions by consistently practicing the Feldenkrais method.

The label of failure is, after all, only a label. If we select and attack it, we can also remove and replace it. Labels should accurately represent their products, and the label of failure is certainly not a true representation of our inner worth and abilities.

Most of us have known people who were labeled failures in life simply because they did not live up to the expectations of others. Yet the norms by which such men and women were valued centered on external rather than internal qualities. The famous schoolteacher Mr. Chips, though judged ineffectual by his peers, was revered and loved by the students he inspired. I believe there may be many modern counterparts of St. Therese of Lisieux, whose "way of love" attracted no fanfare, brought no applause, accomplished no outstanding feats, but brought to others a renewed sense of self-worth and renewed courage to face the challenges of life. People such as these help us redefine our concepts of success and failure.

A new definition of failure and a dedication to perseverance can produce an expansion of our abilities and new feelings of inner power and accomplishment. Failure can be transformed from a disaster into a series of stepping stones leading us to greater feelings

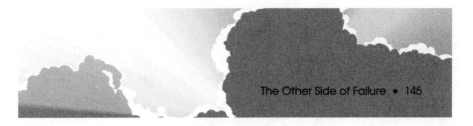

of competence and confidence. Often these feelings are accompanied by a growing desire to share our gifts with others. The circle of love and giving is then complete.

Failure can be a tough label to remove, but it does not have to be. Once we take away the adhesive elements of disaster and permanence, once we know that it is never too late to alter our experience or change our definitions, the label tends to fall off by itself. The choice to act rather than to weep or complain can turn the failure into the beginning of accomplishment and satisfaction.

Hugh Prather, in *Notes to Myself,* says it well:

If I had only...
forgotten future greatness
and looked at the green things and the buildings
and reached out to those around me
and smelled the air
and ignored the forms and self-styled obligations
and heard the rain on the roof and put my arms around my wife
...and it's not too late.

CHAPTER NINETEEN

# *Which Road to Survival?*

A former prisoner of war in Vietnam was asked, "How did you survive with your sanity intact?" His answer was, "You do what you have to do."

I thought about his answer. Like a familiar song it kept coming back to me. Like background music, it accompanied me as I faced my own current challenges, or listened to clients describing theirs.

You do what you have to do.

Not what you think you ought to do, or what someone else tells you is best for you to do. Not what would be the most pleasant thing to do, nor the easiest. You do what the situation demands at this moment. You listen to an inner voice that enables you to act. We are not talking about what to do in the best of all possible situations, we are talking about survival, *now.*

If there is one aspect of survival that emerges from the stories of people who have survived it is the fact that there is no single path for everyone. There are many roads and the choice must be an individual one, based on the circumstances.

Ruth Gordon, speaking to a group of aspiring young actors, focused on persistence and patience. As one who had survived the struggles of many years to find her niche in the theatre, she told her audience "Don't give up!" Ruth knew what she was talking about. For years she was rejected by casting directors because she was too short and too inexperienced. She was not pretty enough or sexy enough. Although the rejections hurt, Ruth believed genuinely that she had talent and would one day be a success. She refused to give up.

Haing Ngor is another person who survived by not giving up. Imprisoned in Cambodia, tortured, forced to watch his loved ones die, he kept the tiny flame of faith alive. When he was able to come to the United States, he was invited to act in a film that told a story similar to his, *The Killing Fields.* Today he travels the world, informing others of the plight of Asian peoples and inspiring them with his own record of courage. His emphasis is on not giving up, no matter how great the trial, and he is an eloquent witness to the merit of this path to survival.

Holding on, refusing to give up, is for many people the road that leads to a new life. But for others, the way is that of surrendering control, of letting go of rigid notions and old beliefs. When this group speaks of "doing what you have to do" they talk about the need to abandon the easy and familiar way, the band-aid solution, the security of tradition. They speak of the need to step into the dark night of new risks.

George Ritchie, in *Return from Tomorrow,* tells about such a man. He was a prisoner in a German concentration camp who became aware that his survival depended on letting go of his hatred. After his wife and children had been killed he made a choice. He states, "I had to decide whether to let myself hate the soldier who had done this...Hate had just killed the six people who mattered most to me in the world. I decided I would spend the rest of my life...loving every person I came in contact with." In that moment of choice came another powerful awakening. He discovered that survival was more than merely staying alive. It meant *prevailing over his inner emotions* as well as the external situation.

At times we all find ourselves in situations which we cannot change, with inner feelings of fear or anger that we cannot immediately banish. Survival means learning to function despite these factors. Virginia Satir expresses it well: "The event does not determine my reaction to the event." In recent years noted physicians and researchers have documented hundreds of cases of people who, though once declared terminal, prevailed over their illnesses. One such patient described his process of healing by saying, "I was dying. Then I not only made the choice to fight for life, but I also made the choice to release my old resentments and to forgive everyone who had hurt me. That's when my real healing began."

The realization: "I have a choice" is itself a powerful source of renewed inner strength. For a person who is struggling to survive, the awareness of being able to control one aspect of life, of not being totally dependent upon the choices of others, can have great impact. It can move us to listen, really listen, to our own inner wisdom in order to make the choice that is best for us at that moment.

The phrase "at that moment" is most important. There is no

magic choice that suits all people at all times. At one moment we may choose to hold on, at another, to let go. We might choose to act swiftly or to wait. Any of these can be proper responses, and all of them might be good choices for us at different moments.

Our ability to hear this inner voice and to trust it increases as we open our ears and our creative imaginations. This voice seems to speak to us through our right-brain activity rather than by a process of logical analysis. Carl Rogers liked to recall his youth on the family farm. There he learned to prevail over the environment by developing a kind of sixth sense. It told him when to plant, how to judge the time for harvesting the wheat before the rains came, how to repair machinery when no repairman was available. This was another case of "doing what you have to do" in order to survive, and of discovering that the power to make good choices resides in each of us.

Later, as a renowned psychotherapist, he taught others to trust in their own wisdom. He never told any of his clients what they ought to do. By listening to them and reflecting back what he had heard he enabled them to listen to themselves in a new way. Gradually they could expand their vision of the current problem and begin to imagine new possibilities. With his encouragement and unconditional love they came to trust their own inner wisdom and make choices based upon it.

Our ability to make such choices does not imply that the process will be painless or the price cheap. The price for survival is never cheap, but what is the alternative? I think of a remark that my former paper boy made. He and his family had escaped from Vietnam as "boat people." The price they paid to arrange the boat trip was their entire life savings. In one stroke they gave up all their possessions, friends and loved ones, to set forth on the journey, not knowing whether they would be killed by pirates before they arrived at a neutral country.

They wound up in Hawaii, where their youngest boy, unable to speak English, found work delivering papers. I saw him grow from a shy, skinny little boy into a warm, friendly teenager. He liked to practice his English and one day I asked him about the high price his family had to pay to get out of Vietnam. He replied, "Yes, but my father know if we stay Vietnam we die. Better have nothing and be alive as family in Hawaii." I could not argue with his reasoning. Even though the price was high, there can be no doubt that it was worth paying.

There is another factor that survivors consistently talk about when they discuss their struggles .It is faith—a basic belief in the positive outcome, an inner conviction that "somehow I will prevail." Unlike other virtues which need the light of understanding, faith is able to flourish in the dark. It can thrive while engaging in combat with doubt and discouragement. Faith can turn the meager resources of a David into weapons that enable us to prevail over the Goliaths of fear and impotence.

With faith we realize that it is "better to light one candle than to curse the darkness." Lighting one candle, taking one step, confronting the needs of one moment, and then of one day—this is the heritage of those who have survived. From early missionaries to pioneering ancestors, faith was the sustaining force that brought them through the darkness to the light of new discoveries.

There is no more eloquent description of the kind of faith that remains alive even during the darkest night of the soul than this message scratched upon the wall of a German home by one of the victims of Nazi persecution:

I believe in the sun—even when it does not shine
I believe in love—even when it is not shown
I believe in God—even when He does not speak.

I saw another example of the same kind of faith and courage when I visited the concentration camp of Mauthausen in Austria. Although the camp had been cleaned and re-painted, I felt a chill beyond that of the cool autumn weather. No amount of paint could eradicate the unspeakable horrors that had taken place within the confines of those gray-walled rooms. In the crematorium, however, I was struck by the sight of a bouquet of flowers, still fresh, placed at the base of one of the giant ovens. There was a note, in Polish, accompanying the flowers. My guide translated it for me:

*It is with deep joy that after twenty-five years, we have been able to make this pilgrimage to the place where our son died. His sacrifice enabled us to survive the death camp and we have returned to honor his memory. His body was destroyed but he never surrendered his faith or his honor. His spirit will live forever in our hearts.*

I was deeply moved by that note, especially when I thought of the pain of these aged parents whose only concern at that moment was to share their love and pride in the son who had given them life.

One final experience in that camp has remained alive for me because of its powerful symbolism. Even today it reminds me of the ever-present possibility of triumphing over life-threatening challenges. Upon leaving the crematorium I looked up at its tall furnace towers and was amazed to see that, despite their height, lack of proper nourishment or adequate light, a slim poplar tree had grown and was swaying gently in the wind.

Searching the ground nearby I found a small, pale green leaf from that tree. I pressed the leaf in a book and brought it home with me. It is on the desk as I write these words. Though the leaf is dry and its colors are now mixtures of rust and brown, for me it remains an inspiring symbol of survival. It reminds me that, despite my current challenges and obstacles, I can prevail. I can choose those things that will ensure my survival.

You do what you have to do. You make the choice to hold on, to let go, to keep believing. And you trust the inner wisdom that guides

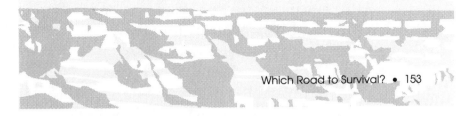

your choice. After that, it is a matter of setting forth on your chosen path, one step at a time, lighting one candle, accepting the support you need to move into the darkness. This is the pattern for prevailing, for thinking beyond survival, for arriving at a place of freedom, safety, and the chance for new beginnings. This self-renewing choice promises the joy of seeing green shoots growing where once there was only a wasteland.

## Intuition Workout by Nancy Rosanoff

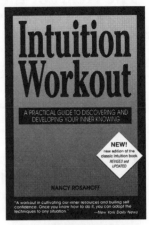

This practical training manual teaches simple techniques to access our deepest sources of inner knowing in any situation.

The author, one of America's outstanding corporate trainers, shows that intuition, like a muscle, is strengthened by training. She outlines dozens of case histories and step-by-step exercises proven effective even with "non-intuitive" people.

"A workout in cultivating our inner resources and building self-confidence. Once you know how to do it, you can adapt the techniques to any situation."
—*New York Daily News*

*Available as a book or audio tape.*
*Also sold as a set for a $3 discount*

**$10.95**

## Your Body Believes Every Word You Say by Barbara Levine

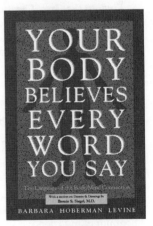

This is the first book to describe the language of the link between mind and body. Barbara Levine's fifteen-year battle with a huge brain tumor led her to trace common phrases like "that breaks my heart" and "it's a pain in the butt" back to the underlying beliefs on which they are based and the symptoms they cause. She lists hundreds of common examples of words we use unconsciously every day, and shows how these "seedthoughts" can set us up for illness.

"Barbara Levine's journey is one of courage and growth. We can all learn from her experience. She shows us what we are capable of and how to achieve our full healing potential."　　　　　　　　—*Bernie Siegel, M.D.*

**$11.95**

## Personal Power Cards by Barbara Gress

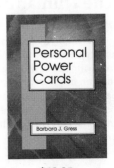

*Personal Power Cards* is a simple, easy to use set of flash cards for emotional wellness. Each set includes 55 cards, a carrying pouch, and an 80 page booklet. The Cards help retrain your feelings to be positive and healthy. Their combination of colors, shapes, and words allows positive thoughts to penetrate deep into your subconscious, "programming" your emotions for health.

"In the twenty years I have been using color and mind imagery with patients, I have never seen any approach have such a great benefit on self-discipline and self-esteem."

—Richard Shames, M.D., Family Practitioner and author of *Healing with Mind Power*

**$18.95**

# The Heart of the Healer
### Edited by Dawson Church & Dr. Alan Sherr

A collection of outstanding personalities on the leading edge of conventional and holistic medicine, including Bernie Siegel, Norman Cousins and Prince Charles, draw on their deepest personal experiences to explore how we get in touch with the essence of wellness. This classic has been called "Exceptional" —*SSC Booknews;* "Thought-provoking" —*Publisher's Weekly;* "Profound...provocative" —*Ram Dass.*

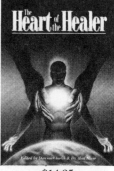

$14.95

# Finding the Great Creative You
### by Lynne Garnett, Ph.D.

"The 90s find more and more people weighing self-employment, 'intrapreneurship,' work-share, and other alternatives to the conventional nine-to-five job. We are demanding that work be a reflection of our creativity, that it be a part of a fulfilled life and not an exception to it.

*Finding the Great Creative You* is an outstanding book in a crowded field. Though light and funny, it is an excel-lent primer on how to approach work in a way appropriate to the next decade, not the last one"

—*Network Magazine*

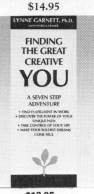

$10.95

# Love Is a Secret
### by Andrew Vidich

What is God's love and how do we experience it? Drawing on the words of saints and scholars from a rich variety of religious traditions, from Taoism to Christianity, from Sufism to Judaism, this book illuminates the psychology of humankind's deepest spiritual experiences.

"In a world yearning to find its unity and connectedness, this book invokes for all to hear, 'Love has only a beginning, my friend; it has no ending.' "

—*Dr. Arthur Stein, Professor Peace Studies, Univ. of R.I.*

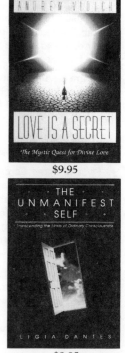

$9.95

# The Unmanifest Self
### by Ligia Dantes

This book, like a warm, gentle friend, guides us toward an experience of self-transformation that is quite different from our usual waking consciousness, and vastly more than an improved version of the old self. *The Unmanifest Self* teaches us the art of objective self-observation, a powerful tool to separate the essential truth of who we are from the labyrinth of thoughts and emotions in which we are often caught.

"...beautiful and inspiring."                    —*Willis Harmon*

$9.95

# Order Form

**(Please print legibly)**                                    Date _____

Name _____

Address _____

City _____ State _____ Zip _____

Phone _____

**Please send a catalog to my friend:**

Name _____

Address _____

City _____ State _____ Zip _____

**Quantity Discounts!**

**$2 off if you order 2 items**
**$3 off if you order 3 items**
**$4 off if you order 4 items, etc...**

| Item | Qty. | Price | Amount |
|------|------|-------|--------|
| Intuition Workout (book) *Second Edition* | | $10.95 | |
| Intuition Workout (tape) | | $9.95 | |
| Your Body Believes Every Word You Say | | $11.95 | |
| Personal Power Cards | | $18.95 | |
| The Heart of the Healer | | $14.95 | |
| Finding the Great Creative You | | $10.95 | |
| Love is a Secret | | $9.95 | |
| The Unmanifest Self | | $9.95 | |
| | | Subtotal | |
| | | Quantity Discount | |
| | Calif. res. add 8.25% sales tax | | |
| | | Shipping | |
| | | Grand Total | |

**Add for shipping:**
Book Rate: $2.50 for first item, $1.50 for ea. add. item
First Class/UPS: $4.00 for first item, $2.00 ea. add. item
Canada/Mexico: One-and-a-half times shipping rates.
Overseas: Double shipping rates.

**Check type of payment:**

☐ Check or money order enclosed

☐ VISA   ☐ MasterCard

Acct. # _____

Exp. Date _____

Signature _____

Send order to:

**Aslan Publishing**
**PO Box 108**
**Lower Lake, CA 95457**

or call to order:
**(707) 995-3906**
**(800) 275-2606**

GR

# Order Form

**(Please print legibly)**                         Date _____

Name _____

Address _____

City _____ State _____ Zip _____

Phone _____

**Please send a catalog to my friend:**

Name _____

Address _____

City _____ State _____ Zip _____

**Quantity Discounts!**

**$2 off if you order 2 items**
**$3 off if you order 3 items**
**$4 off if you order 4 items, etc...**

| Item | Qty. | Price | Amount |
|------|------|-------|--------|
| Intuition Workout (book) *Second Edition* | | $10.95 | |
| Intuition Workout (tape) | | $9.95 | |
| Your Body Believes Every Word You Say | | $11.95 | |
| Personal Power Cards | | $18.95 | |
| The Heart of the Healer | | $14.95 | |
| Finding the Great Creative You | | $10.95 | |
| Love is a Secret | | $9.95 | |
| The Unmanifest Self | | $9.95 | |
| | | Subtotal | |
| | | Quantity Discount | |
| | Calif. res. add 8.25% sales tax | | |
| | | Shipping | |
| | | Grand Total | |

**Add for shipping:**
Book Rate: $2.50 for first item, $1.50 for ea. add. item
First Class/UPS: $4.00 for first item, $2.00 ea. add. item
Canada/Mexico: One-and-a-half times shipping rates.
Overseas: Double shipping rates.

**Check type of payment:**

☐ Check or money order enclosed

☐ VISA    ☐ MasterCard

Acct. # _____

Exp. Date _____

Signature _____

Send order to:
**Aslan Publishing**
**PO Box 108**
**Lower Lake, CA  95457**

or call to order:
**(707) 995-3906**
**(800) 275-2606**